Rare Diseases of the Immune System

Series Editors: Lorenzo Emmi, Domenico Prisco

According to the European Parliament, a disease is considered rare when it affects no more than 5 out of 10,000 people. People with rare diseases are not that scarce, however, since we are talking about a phenomenon that affects hundreds of thousands of people in Italy and several millions all over Europe. Many associations, both national and international, have been created in recent years to inform and safeguard patients affected by these syndromes. At the same time, across various disciplines the medical and scientific awareness of the challenges posed by these diseases has risen inexorably. Rare diseases due to alterations in the immune system represent a field of medical science of great interest that is undergoing continuous expansion; these syndromes have a great social and economic impact because they often affect young or very young people at the height of their social activities and relationships. In recent years, much information has been acquired on pathogenesis, diagnosis, and therapy, allowing us to confront these syndromes in a more holistic manner. The series editors are acknowledged experts on immune diseases who have published extensively on various facets of this branch of medicine. This series will be an invaluable resource for immunologists, rheumatologists, hematologists and medical practitioners looking to update their knowledge and a useful educational tool for residents and students.

Indexed in Scopus

Interested authors should contact the corresponding series editor, Lorenzo Emmi at: lorenzoemmi@yahoo.it

Mario Milco D'Elios
Editor

Severe Combined Immunodeficiency

Springer

Editor
Mario Milco D'Elios
Department of Molecular and Developmental Medicine
University of Siena
Siena, Italy

ISSN 2282-6505 ISSN 2283-6403 (electronic)
Rare Diseases of the Immune System
ISBN 978-3-031-78863-5 ISBN 978-3-031-78864-2 (eBook)
https://doi.org/10.1007/978-3-031-78864-2

This Springer imprint is published by the registered company Springer Nature Switzerland AG
The registered company address is: Gewerbestrasse 11, 6330 Cham, Switzerland

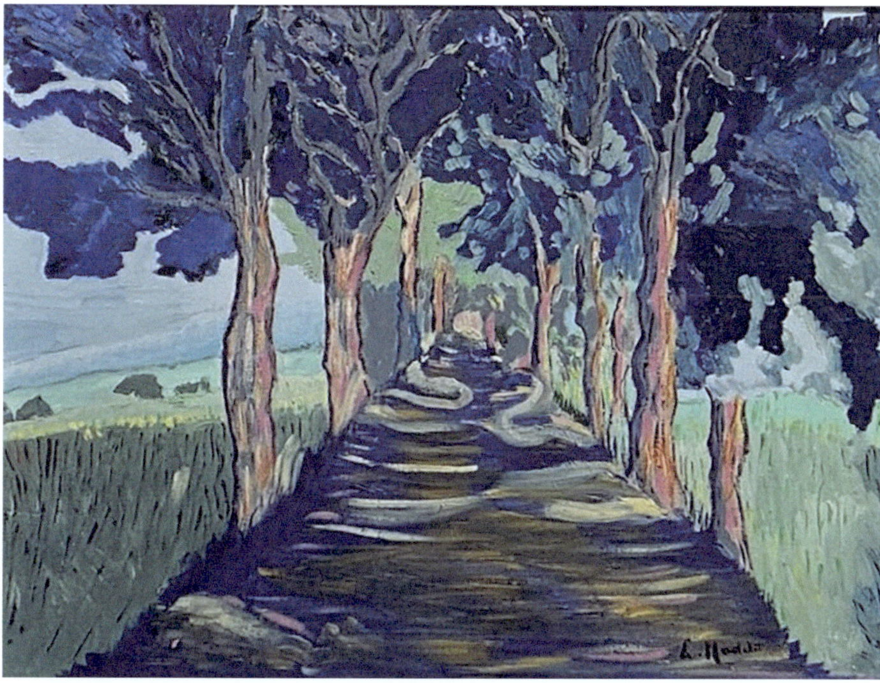

Preface

Severe combined immunodeficiency (SCID) is the most severe primary immune deficiency, consisting of a heterogeneous group of genetic defects affecting the immune system development and function. The overall frequency is estimated to 1 in 40,000–75,000 newborns and despite it is a prenatal disorder, frequently SCID is observed in the first few months of life and the median age at diagnosis is 4–7 months. SCID is a category of inborn errors of immunity (IEI) characterized by absence of both T and B lymphocytes function, resulting in life-threatening susceptibility to infections. The curative treatment for SCID is allogenic hematopoietic stem cells transplant (HSCT). An HLA-matched related donor is the preferred option for the transplant, with survival rates reaching up to 90%. Alternative options include matched unrelated donors, haploidentical parents, mismatched related donors, or cord blood donors. The latest guidelines recommend conditioning prior to HSCT, with the optimal conditioning strategy being tailored to each patient based on their specific genetic defect.

The clinical, molecular, and bioinformatic aspects of SCID are here described in detail. This volume provides an overview of systemic and mucosal immune responses and describes how dysfunctional immune responses underlie the pathogenesis of SCID.

The awareness of SCID has highly increased in the past years, thanks to the creation of international registries and associations devoted to primary immunodeficiencies (PID), such as the European Societies for Immunodeficiencies (ESID), the Foundation for Primary Immunodeficiencies (FPID), the International Patient Organization for Primary Immunodeficiencies (IPOPI), the Latin America Society for Immunodeficiencies (LASID), the Australasian Society of Clinical Immunology and Allergy PID Register, the Immune Deficiencies Foundation Australia (IFSA), the Japanese Society for Immunodeficiency and Autoinflammatory Diseases (JSIAD), the Asian Pacific Society for Immunodeficiency (APSID), and the African Society for Immunodeficiencies (ASID), due to both patient advocacy and research discoveries.

Chapter 2 describes the large panel of genetic defects associated with severe combined immune deficiency and their impact on lymphocyte development. SCID is characterized by defective T lymphocyte development, in some cases associated with a defect in either B lymphocyte or natural killer cell (NK) development. The characterization of gene defects in SCID and the associated clinical phenotypes have important implications in the diagnosis and the therapeutic management of SCID patients.

Chapter 3 focuses on bioinformatics in PID leading the reader towards the *computational immunology* era. *Computational immunology* uses bioinformatics tools to transform immunology datasets into computationally accessible information, contributing significantly to the field. The chapter provides a concise description of the most frequently applied algorithms for B and T cell receptor structural prediction and explains how the integration of multi-omics approaches, including single-cell RNA sequencing, metagenomics, proteomics, and metabolomics, leads to new diagnostics, biomarkers discovery, as well as novel therapies. This chapter highlights the important role of artificial intelligence and machine learning for the detection of PID.

Chapter 4 provides a comprehensive guide to the clinical management of patients with SCID and describes all the diagnostic tools and the therapeutic approaches. The outcome of HSCT therapy of SCID is strongly influenced by the patient's age and infectious status. Early diagnosis and a multidisciplinary approach are crucial to bridge these patients to transplant in the best possible condition. Infection prevention strategies, including antimicrobial prophylaxis against bacteria, viruses, and fungi, immunoglobulin replacement therapy, and strict isolation measures, must be implemented. While live attenuated vaccines are contraindicated, killed and microbial subcomponent vaccines can be safely administered. Gene therapy is also emerging as a safe alternative to allogeneic HSCT for specific genetic conditions causing SCID, such as Adenosine Deaminase Deficiency (ADA)-SCID.

The aim of Chap. 6 is to highlight that late-onset combined-immunodeficiency (LOCID), caused by variants in the same genes usually associated with classical SCID, may affect patients beyond typical SCID found in infancy. The main mechanisms responsible for atypical SCID presentations are hypomorphic variants, mosaicism, and somatic reversion. Hypomorphic variants reduce the quantity or stability of mRNA or protein or result in functional defects. The delayed presentations of LOCID can be very challenging both for the diagnosis and for the clinical management of patients affected.

We hope that this book focused on the universe of SCID will boost the curiosity of young students on PID and the immune system, as well the interest of MD specialists in clinical immunology, pediatricians, hematologists, gastroenterologists, and scientists all over the world.

Siena, Italy
30 September 2024

Mario Milco D'Elios

Contents

1 **Mucosal Immunity in Primary Immunodeficiencies** 1
Sofia D'Elios, Marisa Benagiano, Evangelina Asvestopoulou, Mario Milco D'Elios, and Chiara Della Bella

2 **Genetic Defects Associated with SCID and Their Impact on Lymphocyte Development** 11
Nagaja Capitani and Cosima Tatiana Baldari

3 **Bioinformatics in Primary Immunodeficiencies: Towards a "Computational Immunology" Era** 23
Josefina del Pilar Martínez Vásquez and Alexios-Fotios Mentis

4 **Clinical Management of Severe Combined Immunodeficiencies** 67
Francesco Pegoraro, Marta Voarino, and Eleonora Gambineri

5 **Hot Topics in Severe Combined Immunodeficiency (SCID)** 79
Sofia D'Elios, Mario Milco D'Elios, and Nagaja Capitani

6 **Late-Onset and Hypomorphic Presentation of Severe Combined Immune Deficiency** 91
Lorenzo Salvati, Boaz Palterer, and Lorenzo Cosmi

7 **Gut Involvement in Cellular Immunodeficiencies** 103
Sofia D'Elios, Marisa Benagiano, Evangelina Asvestopoulou, Mario Milco D'Elios, and Chiara Della Bella

Index 119

Mucosal Immunity in Primary Immunodeficiencies

1

Sofia D'Elios, Marisa Benagiano, Evangelina Asvestopoulou, Mario Milco D'Elios, and Chiara Della Bella

1.1 The MALT

The mucosa-associated lymphoid tissue (MALT) is a secondary lymphoid organ consisting of more or less organized lymphoid structures [1]. It comprises various subregions, with the most significant ones being the gut-associated lymphoid tissue (GALT), nasal-associated lymphoid tissue (NALT), and bronchus-associated lymphoid tissue (BALT). In the adult human airway, there is no evidence of organized lymphoid tissue under normal conditions, but induced bronchus-associated lymphoid tissue (iBALT) can be observed in pathological states. MALT exhibits region-specific inductive and effector sites. The systemic and mucosal immune systems possess distinct functional structures and can be independently activated and regulated [2, 3]. Key features of MALT include the presence of diverse cell types like B cells, T cells, dendritic cells (DC), and innate immune cells, working collaboratively to mount an effective immune response. Additionally, MALT shares common traits such as the absence of afferent lymphatics and the presence of high endothelial regions [1, 4, 5].

This chapter is partially based on the chapter published in the book: Cellular Primary Immunodeficiencies, Springer, 2021, edited by Mario Milco D'Elios, Cosima Tatiana Baldari, Francesco Annunziato.

S. D'Elios
Department of Clinical and Experimental Medicine, University of Pisa, Pisa, Italy

M. Benagiano
Department of Experimental and Clinical Medicine, University of Florence, Florence, Italy

E. Asvestopoulou · M. M. D'Elios (✉) · C. Della Bella
Department of Molecular and Developmental Medicine, University of Siena, Siena, Italy
e-mail: delios@unisi.it

M. M. D'Elios (ed.), *Severe Combined Immunodeficiency*, Rare Diseases of the Immune System, https://doi.org/10.1007/978-3-031-78864-2_1

1.2 Epithelia and Innate Mucosal Immunity in Respiratory Tract and Gut

Mucosal epithelia are consistently exposed to external antigens, collaborating with various cell types to safeguard the gastrointestinal and respiratory tracts [6]. The airway epithelium plays a pivotal role in regulating the secretion and composition of saliva, encompassing mucus, secretory immunoglobulin A (SIgA), and humoral innate immune proteins like lactoferrin, lysozyme, and defensins. This regulation establishes a physical and chemical barrier, preventing infections and potential chronic inflammatory processes resulting from continual antigen exposure. The mucosal epithelium, working alongside localized antigen-presenting cells, is crucial in bridging the innate and adaptive immune systems by producing cytokines and chemokines, initiating inflammation during infections. Nevertheless, specialized lymphoid cells and immune mechanisms at mucosal sites play an immunosuppressive role in adaptive immune processes, tightly modulating and controlling inflammatory responses. L-selectin, prominently present in the head and neck mucosa and lymph nodes, governs the trafficking of lymphocytes to these sites. α-defensins regulate the mucosal immune system in the gut, averting microbial invasion at the epithelial surface and modulating the activity of diverse T cell subpopulations for subsequent adaptive responses [7, 8]. Increasing data indicate that at the mucosal level, innate immunity primarily regulates the immune response [9]. Congenital defects in the epithelium can lead to early-onset inflammatory bowel disease (IBD) [10]. The epithelium plays a crucial regulatory role in innate immunity. Severe colitis has been observed in two children with biallelic loss-of-function mutation in the *ALPI* gene, which codes for intestinal phosphatase alkaline—a brush border metalloenzyme that hydrolyzes phosphate from the lipid A moiety of lipopolysaccharides, thereby significantly reducing Toll-like receptor 4 agonist activity [11].

Mutations in TTC7A, an epithelial protein, can lead to various phenotypes, some of which may be associated with combined immunodeficiency (CID), such as multiple intestinal atresia (MIA) and very early-onset inflammatory bowel disease [12].

The intestinal epithelium's expression of antimicrobial peptides is believed to play a crucial role in controlling bacterial levels around epithelial cells and has recently been proposed to be a key factor in the pathogenesis of inflammatory bowel disease. The NF-κB signaling pathway is instrumental in regulating the expression of antimicrobial peptides [13].

The absence of defensins has been implicated in the development of colitis in the context of NEMO hypomorphic mutation. In $NEMO^{IEC\text{-}KO}$ mice, the expression of beta-defensin-3 (homologous to human beta-defensin-2, associated with colonic Crohn's disease in humans) [14] was significantly downregulated [15].

1.3 Mucosal T Cells

Conventional T cells undergo development in the thymus starting from double-negative ($CD4^-CD8^-$) progenitors. Following TCRβ expression, $CD4^-$ $CD8^-$ cells progress to a double-positive ($CD4^+CD8^+$) stage. Through negative selection, strongly self-reactive cells are eliminated, while T cells with low affinity to self-antigens develop into single-positive $CD4^+$ (via interaction with MHC II) and single-positive $CD8^+$ (through interaction with MHC I) [16].

Upon exiting the thymus, naive $CD4^+$ T and $CD8\alpha\beta^+$ T cells travel through the circulation to gut-associated lymphoid tissues (GALTs), including mesenteric lymph nodes and Peyer's patches. In these locations, they are primed by antigen-presenting cells (APCs) and the upregulation of gut-homing molecules like CCR9, CD44, integrin α4β7, LFA-1, and VLA-4. These molecules enable the T cells to home to various mucosal sites guided by specific ligands. APCs and intestinal epithelial cells (IECs) regulate the differentiation of $CD4^+$ T cells into Th1, Th2, Th17, and intestinal Treg (iTreg) in response to diverse food or microbial antigens present at the site [17]. These intestinal T cells predominantly migrate to the lamina propria and exhibit an effector memory phenotype.

A small subset of thymocytes, not subject to thymic selection, lacks the conventional T cell coreceptors (CD4 and CD8αβ) and expresses either TCRγδ or TCRαβ and CD8αα homodimers. These unconventional T cells mainly serve regulatory functions and are primarily located between the gut lumen and enterocytes as intraepithelial lymphocytes (IELs) [18–21].

γδ T cells have also been identified in the lung during respiratory infections, contributing to the clearance of intracellular and extracellular bacteria. In cases of active pulmonary tuberculosis, circulating γδ T cells play a crucial role as a significant source of IL17 [22, 23].

Both conventional and nonconventional T cells collaborate to provide protection against pathogens while simultaneously maintaining immune tolerance to commensals and antigens derived from food, thereby contributing to intestinal homeostasis. In this context, intraepithelial lymphocytes (IELs) play a crucial role in preserving the barrier function of the gut. The mucosal homeostasis in the gut relies on a delicate balance between T cells with effector functions, which swiftly initiate an immune response against pathogens, and regulatory T cells, including IL-10-producing $CD4^+$ T cells. Any imbalance among these specialized components of the adaptive immune system has the potential to lead to autoimmune enteropathy. Notably, IELs have been identified in the lung as well. In biopsies from healthy volunteers, approximately 20 bronchial IELs per 100 epithelial cell nuclei were observed, predominantly expressing ab T cell receptors [24].

Intestinal tolerance to commensal microorganisms and food primarily relies on $FOXP3^+$ Treg cells. Of the total $CD4^+$ T cells in the intestine, approximately 30% are situated in the colon, with about 20% of those in the small intestine. The presence and activity of Treg cells are influenced by the gut microbiota. In a mouse model, germ-free mice exhibited a significant reduction in the number of Treg cells in the small intestine, indicating a microbiota-independent induction in the small intestine but not in the colon [25].

Similarly, the airway mucosa hosts specialized lymphoid cells that regulate and modulate inflammatory responses. Studies have revealed that inducible Tregs (foxp3^{+}helios^{-}) in the airways exhibit the highest frequency of IL-17-producing cells among CD4^{+} T cell subsets. Additionally, a greater percentage of foxp3^{-}CD4^{+} T cells in the airways produce IL-10 compared to peripheral blood [26]. The heightened frequency of inducible Tregs producing IL-17 may play a crucial role in facilitating the transport of secretory immunoglobulin A (SIgA) by inducing T helper (Th) 17 cells, as demonstrated in Peyer's patches, which is essential for T cell-dependent immunoglobulin A production [27].

MAIT (Mucosal-Associated Invariant T) cells, classified as nonconventional T cell subsets, display distinctive features. Unlike conventional T cells, when MAIT cells emerge from the thymus, they already possess the capability to function as effector cells. However, their T cell receptors (TCRs) exhibit limitations in recognizing a broad spectrum of antigens. These unique characteristics position MAIT cells in a role that bridges the gap between the innate and adaptive immune systems.

MAIT cells are distributed in mucosal tissues, including the intestine, lung, and liver. These cells specifically recognize conserved nonpeptide antigens presented by the MHC class I-like protein MR1. Upon activation, they produce TNF-α and IFN-γ, playing a crucial role in controlling bacterial intracellular infections. In the lung, MAIT cells are particularly significant in respiratory infections. The circulation of MAIT cells is reduced in tuberculosis patients and almost absent in those with active tuberculosis, likely due to their recruitment to the lung. In murine models of respiratory bacterial infections, these cells were observed to expand and produce IFN-γ, TNF-α, and IL-17. Mice lacking MAIT cells exhibited a diminished and delayed response to BCG and *F. tularensis* infection [28, 29]. Recent findings indicate alterations in MAIT cells in CVID (Common Variable Immunodeficiency) patients, with a reduction in both number and frequency [30]. The remaining cells expressed activation markers and exhibited a reduced IFN-γ response when challenged in vitro with *E. coli*, similarly to patients affected by chronic infections like HIV, HTLV1, and HCV [31–34], and to patients with cystic fibrosis [35]. Additionally, lower blood MAIT cell levels were observed in patients with chronic *H. pylori* or mycobacterial infections [36, 37] (Fig. 1.1).

1.3.1 Autoimmune Enteropathy, Regulatory T Cells, and IL-17 Production

Autoimmune enteropathy (AIE) is a rare condition clinically characterized by chronic diarrhea and malabsorption, often associated with autoimmune comorbidities [38].

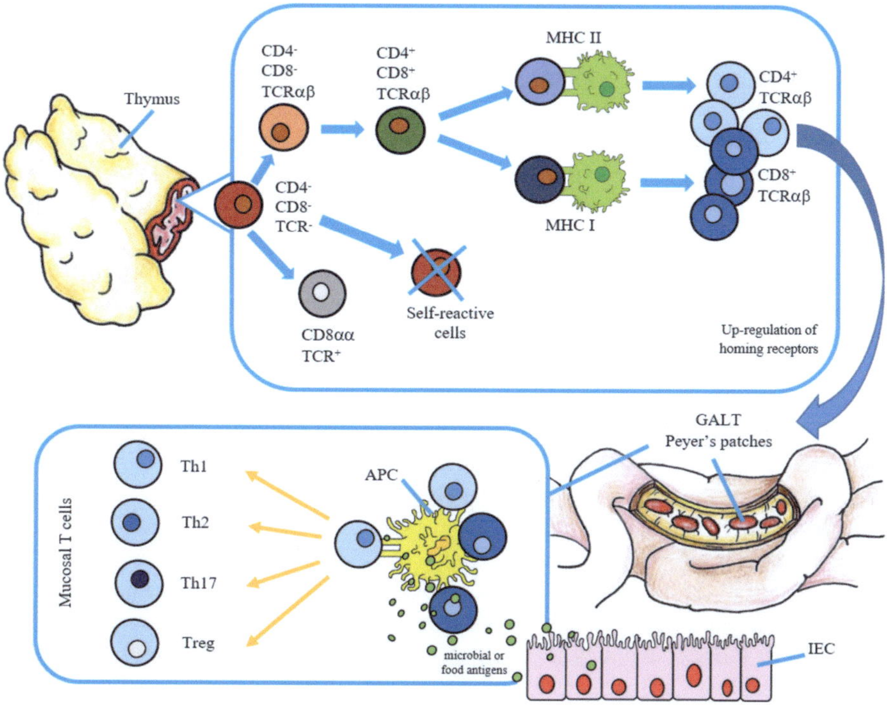

Fig. 1.1 Origin and development of T lymphocyte lineage subsets. Conventional T cells originate from double-negative ($CD4^-CD8^-$) precursors in the thymus. Upon TCRαβ expression, $CD4^-CD8^-$ cells progress to a double-positive ($CD4^+CD8^+$) stage. Strongly self-reactive cells undergo negative selection, while those with low affinity to self-antigens develop into single-positive $CD4^+$ (through interaction with MHC II) and single-positive $CD8^+$ (via interaction with MHC I). Upon thymic egress, naïve $CD4^+\alpha\beta^+$ T and $CD8^+\alpha\beta^+$ T cells travel through the bloodstream to gut-associated lymphoid tissues, such as mesenteric lymph nodes and Peyer's patches. In these sites, they are primed by antigen-presenting cells (APCs) and upregulate gut-homing molecules like CCR9, CD44, integrin α4β7, LFA-1, and VLA-4, allowing them to home to various mucosal sites guided by specific ligands. APCs and intestinal epithelial cells (IECs) regulate the differentiation of $CD4^+$ T cells into Th1-producing IFN-γ, Th2-producing IL-4, Th17-producing IL-17, and intestinal T regulatory cells (Treg) in response to microbial or food antigens. These mucosal T cells predominantly migrate to the lamina propria and exhibit an effector memory phenotype. A small subset of thymocytes bypass thymic selection, lacking the typical "conventional" T cell coreceptors. These unconventional T cells, expressing either TCRγδ or TCRαβ and CD8αα homodimers, are characterized by the absence of typical CD4 and CD8αβ coreceptors. Termed intraepithelial lymphocytes, they predominantly reside between the gut lumen and enterocytes. $\gamma\delta^+$ T cells have also been identified in the lungs during respiratory infections, playing a role in clearing intracellular and extracellular bacteria. Both conventional and unconventional T cells collaborate to protect against pathogens while simultaneously maintaining immune tolerance to commensals and antigens from food, actively contributing to intestinal homeostasis

The development of AIE is significantly influenced by an imbalance between regulatory T cells (Tregs) and the activation of effector T cells.

Patients diagnosed with immune dysregulation polyendocrinopathy enteropathy X-linked syndrome (IPEX), an X-linked disorder resulting from mutations in FOXP3, commonly exhibit symptoms of autoimmune enteropathy (AIE). The role of Foxp3 is pivotal for the development and function of regulatory T cells ($CD4^+CD25^+$) [39]. Additionally, cases of adult-onset AIE not associated with IPEX have been documented [40]. In individuals with IPEX, there is a reduction in the expression of both FOXP3 and $CD4^+CD25^+$ regulatory T cells, potentially contributing to intestinal inflammation and villous atrophy due to uncontrolled activation of gut-associated lymphoid tissue. Biopsies from the duodenal mucosa of these patients reveal infiltrates of $CD4^+CD8^+$ T cells [41].

In non-IPEX adult-onset AIE cases, a severe instance demonstrated intraepithelial T lymphocytes (IEL) in the duodenal mucosa producing IFN-γ and IL-17. This cytokine production was absent in samples from Crohn's and celiac disease or healthy controls. The study also revealed that TCR-activated IL-17 production has distinct cytokine and transforming growth factor-β (TGF-β) requirements in lamina propria and intraepithelial $CD4^+$ and $CD8^+$ lymphocytes. Active TGF-β was detected in the intestinal mucosa of AIE patients, with Tregs expressing low FOXP3 maintaining the ability to produce TGF-β and enhancing IL-17 production by IEL $CD8^+$ T cells [42]. Interestingly, in mouse models, Treg cells were found to suppress CD8α+ T cell receptor (TCR)$\gamma\delta^+$ T cells, including an interleukin-17 (IL-17)-expressing population responsible for inflammatory colitis [43].

Defects in regulatory T cells form the basis of gastrointestinal involvement in immune dysregulation syndromes. Gastrointestinal complications may occur in IPEX syndrome, CD25 deficiency, CTLA4 insufficiency, and LRBA deficiency.

An escalated and unregulated activity of effector T cells can also result in inflammatory enteropathy.

The fundamental cause of autoimmune enteropathy in certain complex immune deficiencies, such as MALT1 deficiency and DOCK8 deficiency, lies in an imbalance in Treg/effector T cell activation. In these conditions, a diminished activity of Tregs has been documented. Similarly, the dysregulation in Treg/effector T cell activation is implicated in autoimmune enteropathy associated with STAT1 GOF [44], STAT3 GOF mutations [45], and the recently identified JAK1 GOF mutation [46].

1.3.2 $CD4^+$ T Cell Depletion in Gut Mucosal and Chronic Granulomatous Disease

Chronic granulomatous disease (CGD) is an inherited primary immunodeficiency that impacts phagocytes. Individuals with CGD carry mutations in NADPH oxidase, resulting in impaired production of reactive oxygen species (ROS) by neutrophils and monocytes. This leads to defects in clearing microorganisms and results in chronic inflammation [47, 48]. While T cell alterations have been observed in CGD patients [49], the underlying mechanisms behind these changes remain unclear and require further investigation.

In a case study involving an adult CGD patient, progressive $CD4^+$ lymphopenia was observed, accompanied by a reduction in naive cells, lymphocyte activation, and an expansion of interleukin (IL)-17-producing CD4 T cells. At the age of 34, the patient experienced persistent diarrhea with watery stool, lacking blood or mucous, along with hypoalbuminemia. Despite an absence of identified microbial causes or malabsorption, an endoscopy with biopsies revealed lymphoid aggregates and inflammatory infiltrates. Flow cytometry analysis of cell suspensions from sigmoid biopsies showed a decreased number of $CD4^+$ T cells at the intestinal mucosa level, leading to a reduced $CD4^+/CD8^+$ ratio compared to the control [50, 51].

The pathogenesis of T cell alterations in the mucosal compartment appears to be linked to immunosenescence, but further investigation is necessary to fully understand these mechanisms.

References

1. D'Elios MM, Rizzi M (2019) Humoral primary immunodeficiencies. Springer, Cham
2. Mei HE, Yoshida T, Sime W, Hiepe F, Thiele K, Manz RA et al (2009) Blood-borne human plasma cells in steady state are derived from mucosal immune responses. Blood 113(11):2461–2469
3. Weitkamp JH, Kallewaard NL, Bowen AL, Lafleur BJ, Greenberg HB, Crowe JE Jr (2005) VH1-46 is the dominant immunoglobulin heavy chain gene segment in rotavirus-specific memory B cells expressing the intestinal homing receptor alpha4beta7. J Immunol 174(6):3454–3460
4. Macpherson AJ, McCoy KD, Johansen FE, Brandtzaeg P (2008) The immune geography of IgA induction and function. Mucosal Immunol 1(1):11–22
5. Dwivedy A, Aich P (2011) Importance of innate mucosal immunity and the promises it holds. Int J Gen Med 4:299–311. https://doi.org/10.2147/IJGM.S17525
6. Weitnauer M, Mijošek V, Dalpke A (2016) Control of local immunity by airway epithelial cells. Mucosal Immunol 9:287–298. https://doi.org/10.1038/mi.2015.126
7. Wilson CL, Ouellette AJ, Satchell DP et al (1999) Regulation of intestinal alpha-defensin activation by the metalloproteinase matrilysin in innate host defense. Science 286(5437):113–117. https://doi.org/10.1126/science.286.5437.113
8. Heather LC, Cole MA, Lygate CA et al (2006) Fatty acid transporter levels and palmitate oxidation rate correlate with ejection fraction in the infarcted rat heart. Cardiovasc Res 72:430–437
9. Heritage PL, Brook MA, Underdown BJ et al (1998) Intranasal immunization with polymer-grafted microparticles activates the nasal-associated lymphoid tissue and draining lymph nodes. Immunology 93:249–256
10. Parlato M, Charbit-Henrion F et al (2017) First identification of biallelic inherited duox2 inactivating mutations as a cause of very early onset inflammatory bowel disease. Gastroenterology 153:609–611.e3
11. Parlato M, Charbit-Henrion F, Pan J et al (2018) Human ALPI deficiency causes inflammatory bowel disease and highlights a key mechanism of gut homeostasis. EMBO Mol Med 10:e8483
12. Jardine S, Dhingani N, Muise AM (2019) TTC7A: steward of intestinal health. Cell Mol Gastroenterol Hepatol 7(3):555–557
13. Wehkamp J, Fellermann K, Herrlinger KR, Bevins CL, Stange EF (2005) Mechanisms of disease: defensins in gastrointestinal diseases. Nat Clin Pract Gastroenterol Hepatol 2:406–415

14. Fellermann K et al (2006) A chromosome 8 gene-cluster polymorphism with low human β-defensin 2 gene copy number predisposes to Crohn disease of the colon. Am J Hum Genet 79:439–448
15. Nenci A, Becker C, Wullaert A et al (2007) Epithelial NEMO links innate immunity to chronic intestinal inflammation. Nature 446:557–561. https://doi.org/10.1038/nature05698
16. Hayday A, Gibbons D (2008) Brokering the peace: the origin of intestinal T cells. Mucosal Immunol 1(3):172–174. https://doi.org/10.1038/mi.2008.8.Brokering
17. Ma H, Tao W, Zhu S (2019) T lymphocytes in the intestinal mucosa: defense and tolerance. Cell Mol Immunol 16(3):216–224. https://doi.org/10.1038/s41423-019-0208-2
18. Baldwin TA, Hogquist KA, Jameson SC (2004) The fourth way? Harnessing aggressive tendencies in the thymus. J Immunol 173(11):6515–6520. https://doi.org/10.4049/jimmunol.173.11.6515
19. Chen Y, Chou K, Fuchs E, Havran WL, Boismenu R (2002) Protection of the intestinal mucosa by intraepithelial γδ T cells. Proc Natl Acad Sci USA 99(22):14338–14343. https://doi.org/10.1073/pnas.212290499
20. Darlington D, Rogers AW (1966) Epithelial lymphocytes in the small intestine of the mouse. J Anat 100(Pt 4):813–830
21. Zeitz M, Schieferdecker HL, Ullrich R, Jahn HU, James SP, Riecken EO (1991) Phenotype and function of lamina propria T lymphocytes. Immunol Res 10(3–4):199–206. https://doi.org/10.1007/BF02919693
22. Wands JM, Roark CL, Aydintug MK, Jin N, Hahn YS et al (2005) Distribution and leukocyte contacts of gammadelta T cells in the lung. J Leukoc Biol 78:1086–1096
23. Peng MY, Wang ZH, Yao CY, Jiang LN, Jin QL et al (2008) Interleukin 17-producing gamma delta T cells increased in patients with active pulmonary tuberculosis. Cell Mol Immunol 5:203–208
24. Fournier M, Lebargy F, Le Roy F, Ladurie LE, Pariente R (1989) Intraepithelial T-lymphocyte subsets in the airways of normal subjects and of patients with chronic bronchitis. Am Rev Respir Dis 140:4737–4742
25. Bilate AM, Lafaille JJ (2012) Induced CD4+Foxp3+ regulatory T cells in immune tolerance. Annu Rev Immunol 30(1):733–758. https://doi.org/10.1146/annurev-immunol-020711-075043
26. Ballke C, Gran E, Baekkevold ES et al (2016) Characterization of regulatory T-cell markers in CD4+ T cells of the upper airway mucosa. PLoS One 11:e0148826. https://doi.org/10.1371/journal.pone.0148826
27. Hirota K, Turner J-E, Villa M et al (2013) Plasticity of Th17 cells in Peyer's patches is responsible for the induction of T cell-dependent IgA responses. Nat Immunol 14:372–379. https://doi.org/10.1038/ni.2552
28. Gold MC, Cerri S, Smyk-Pearson S, Cansler ME, Vogt TM et al (2010) Human mucosal associated invariant T cells detect bacterially infected cells. PLoS Biol 8:e1000407
29. Meierovics A, Yankelevich WJ, Cowley SC (2013) MAIT cells are critical for optimal mucosal immune responses during in vivo pulmonary bacterial infection. Proc Natl Acad Sci USA 110:E3119–E3128
30. Paquin-Proulx D, Santos BAN et al (2017) Loss of circulating mucosal-associated invariant T cells in common variable immunodeficiency is associated with immune activation and loss of eomes and PLZF. ImmunoHorizons 1(7):142–155. https://doi.org/10.4049/immunohorizons.1700039
31. Leeansyah E, Ganesh A, Quigley MF et al (2013) Activation, exhaustion, and persistent decline of the antimicrobial MR1-restricted MAIT-cell population in chronic HIV-1 infection. Blood 121:1124–1135
32. Cosgrove C, Ussher JE, Rauch A et al (2013) Early and nonreversible decrease of CD161++/MAIT cells in HIV infection. Blood 121:951–961
33. Paquin-Proulx D, Greenspun BC, Costa EA et al (2017) MAIT cells are reduced in frequency and functionally impaired in human T lymphotropic virus type 1 infection: potential clinical implications. PLoS One 12:e0175345

34. Hengst J, Strunz B, Deterding K et al (2016) Nonreversible MAIT cell-dysfunction in chronic hepatitis C virus infection despite successful interferon-free therapy. Eur J Immunol 46:2204–2210
35. Smith DJ, Hill GR, Bell SC et al (2014) Reduced mucosal associated invariant T-cells are associated with increased disease severity and Pseudomonas aeruginosa infection in cystic fibrosis. PLoS One 9:e109891
36. Booth JS, Salerno-Goncalves R, Blanchard TG et al (2015) Mucosal-associated invariant T cells in the human gastric mucosa and blood: role in Helicobacter pylori infection. Front Immunol 6:466
37. Kwon YS, Cho YN, Kim MJ et al (2015) Mucosal-associated invariant T cells are numerically and functionally deficient in patients with mycobacterial infection and reflect disease activity. Tuberculosis 95:267–274
38. Gentile NM, Murray JA, Pardi DS (2012) Autoimmune enteropathy: a review and update of clinical management. Curr Gastroenterol Rep 14(5):380–385. https://doi.org/10.1007/s11894-012-0276-2
39. Barzaghi F, Passerini L, Bacchetta R (2012) Immune dysregulation, polyendocrinopathy, enteropathy, X-linked syndrome: a paradigm of immunodeficiency with autoimmunity. Front Immunol 3:1–25. https://doi.org/10.3389/fimmu.2012.00211
40. Moes N, Rieuxlaucat F, Begue B et al (2010) Reduced expression of FOXP3 and regulatory T-cell function in severe forms of early-onset autoimmune enteropathy. Gastroenterology 139(3):770–778. https://doi.org/10.1053/j.gastro.2010.06.006
41. Ruemmele FM, Brousse N, Goulet O (2004) Autoimmune enteropathy: molecular concepts. Curr Opin Gastroenterol 20(6):587–591. https://doi.org/10.1097/00001574-200411000-00014
42. Paroni M, Magarotto A, Tartari S et al (2016) Uncontrolled IL-17 production by intraepithelial lymphocytes in a case of non-IPEX autoimmune enteropathy. Clin Transl Gastroenterol 7(7):e182. https://doi.org/10.1038/ctg.2016.41
43. Park SG, Mathur R, Long M et al (2010) T regulatory cells maintain intestinal homeostasis by suppressing γδ T cells. Immunity 33(5):791–803. https://doi.org/10.1016/j.immuni.2010.10.014
44. Toubiana J, Okada S, Hiller J et al (2016) Heterozygous STAT1 gain-of-function mutations underlie an unexpectedly broad clinical phenotype. Blood 127(25):3154–3164. https://doi.org/10.1182/blood-2015-11-679902
45. Milner JD, Vogel TP, Forbes L et al (2015) Early-onset lymphoproliferation and autoimmunity caused by germline STAT3 gain-of-function mutations. Blood 125(4):591–599. https://doi.org/10.1182/blood-2014-09-602763
46. Gruber CN, Calis JJA, Buta S et al (2020) Complex autoinflammatory syndrome unveils fundamental principles of JAK1 kinase transcriptional and biochemical function. Immunity 53(3):672–684.e11. https://doi.org/10.1016/j.immuni.2020.07.006
47. Di R (2016) Chronic granulomatous disease. Br Med Bull 118(1):50–63. https://doi.org/10.1093/bmb/ldw009
48. Holland SM (2013) Chronic granulomatous disease. Hematol Oncol Clin North Am 27(1):89–99. https://doi.org/10.1016/j.hoc.2012.11.002.Chronic
49. Heltzer M, Jawad AF, Rae J, Curnutte JT, Sullivan KE (2002) Diminished T cell numbers in patients with chronic granulomatous disease. Clin Immunol 105(3):273–278. https://doi.org/10.1006/clim.2002.5291
50. Albuquerque AS, Fernandes SM, Tendeiro R et al (2017) Major CD4 T-cell depletion and immune senescence in a patient with chronic granulomatous disease. Front Immunol 8:4–11. https://doi.org/10.3389/fimmu.2017.00543
51. D'Elios M, Baldari C, Annunziato F (2021) Cellular primary immunodeficiencies. Springer, Cham. https://doi.org/10.1007/978-3-030-70107-9

Genetic Defects Associated with SCID and Their Impact on Lymphocyte Development

2

Nagaja Capitani and Cosima Tatiana Baldari

2.1 Introduction

Severe combined immunodeficiency (SCID) is a group of inherited immune disorders characterized by impaired development and function of T lymphocytes, clinically detectable by the absence or very low number of T cells and defective T-cell function, caused by intrinsic defects in T-cell development [1–3]. Together with the defects affecting the T-cell population, SCID can be variably associated with compromised differentiation of other hematopoietic cell lineages, such as concomitant impairment of B-lymphocyte development and, in some cases, decreased NK cell number and function [4, 5].

2.2 Lymphocyte Development

B and T lymphocytes as well as and natural killer (NK) cells develop starting from a common lymphoid progenitor (CLP). The maturation steps take place mainly in two different specialized microenvironments, the bone marrow (BM) for B and NK cells and the thymus for T cells.

B and T lymphocyte development occurs in ordered steps marked by rearrangement of the antigen receptor genes. The exons which encode B-cell antigen-receptor (BCR)/immunoglobulin (Ig) or T-cell receptor (TCR) variable regions are assembled in developing B or T lymphocytes from germline variable (V), diversity (D), and joining (J) gene segments [6]. The TCRβ chain and BCR/Ig heavy chain (IgH) variable regions are assembled from V, D, and J segments, while TCRα chain and BCR/Ig κ and λ light chain (IgL) regions are assembled from V and J segments [7]

N. Capitani (✉) · C. T. Baldari (✉)
Department of Life Sciences, University of Siena, Siena, Italy
e-mail: capitani2@unisi.it; cosima.baldari@unisi.it

M. M. D'Elios (ed.), *Severe Combined Immunodeficiency*, Rare Diseases of the Immune System, https://doi.org/10.1007/978-3-031-78864-2_2

(Fig. 2.1). Only one gene locus is rearranged at a time, and the loci are each rearranged in a fixed sequence, with the VDJ rearrangements preceding VJ rearrangements. A successful gene rearrangement, termed as "productive" rearrangement, leads to the synthesis of the corresponding product, allowing for progress to the next stage of development.

Together with antigen-receptor rearrangements, lymphocyte development is marked by changes in the expression of other cell-surface and intracellular proteins.

During α:β T lymphocyte development in the thymus, productive VDJ rearrangements lead to expression of the TCRβ chain which assembles with a surrogate TCRα chain to form a pre-TCR on which the subsequent VJ rearrangement leading to the assembly of a mature TCR critically depends. Rearrangements at the TCR loci are accompanied by surface expression of the CD3 complex, the signaling module of the TCR complex, and of the CD4 and CD8 co-receptors. The first step of T-cell development is known as the double-negative (DN) stage, where cells express neither CD4 nor CD8. Two different T-cell lineages originate from these precursors, the γ:δ T cells (not discussed in this chapter), which lack CD4

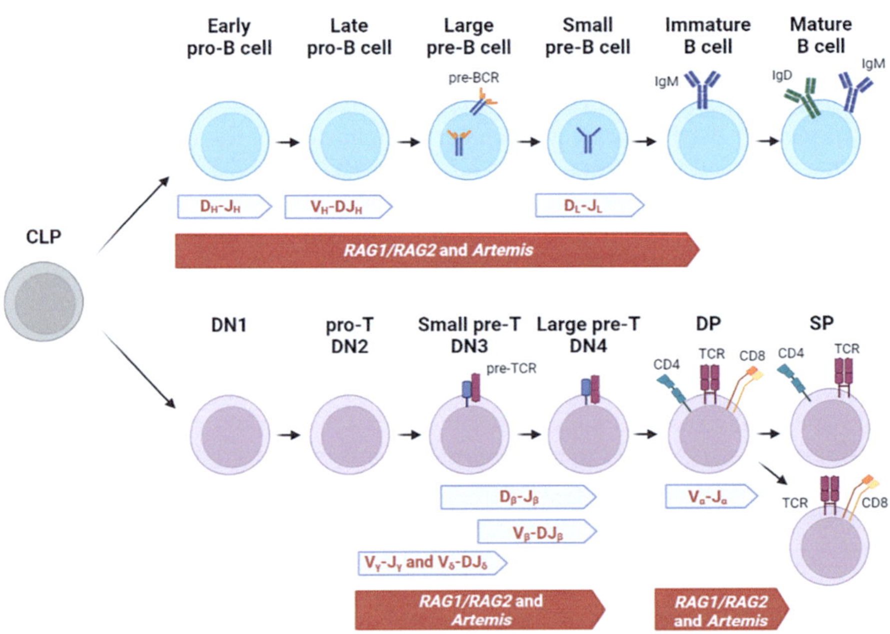

Fig. 2.1 Human B- and T-cell maturation stages. The stages of B cell (top) and T cell (bottom) development are marked by sequential V(D)J recombination events that lead to surface expression of the pre-BCR/BCR in developing B cells, and of the pre-TCR/TCR in thymocytes. Severe forms of SCID characterized by defective T- and B-cell development are caused by mutations in the key components of the recombination machinery, RAG1/2 and Artemis

or CD8 even when mature, and the α:β T cells. The latter continue their development to acquire both CD4 and CD8 expression (double-positive stage, DP). Subsequently, the interaction with self-peptides associated to a major histocompatibility complex (MHC) class I or class II molecules, determines the downregulation of either CD4 or CD8 to produce naïve CD8 or CD4 single positive cells (SP) that, following selection to eliminate self-reactive cells, exit the thymus and circulate to the periphery [8]. There naïve T cells circulate through the blood and lymphatic system until becoming activated in peripheral lymphoid organs by encountering an antigen-presenting cell (APC) bearing an antigenic peptide noncovalently bound to a MHCI or MHCII molecule, recognized by the TCR of CD8 or CD4 T cells, respectively. Following activation, T cells differentiate generating a number of subsets of effector T cells, as well as memory and central memory T cells [9–11].

B-cell lineage development takes place in the BM, where the genes encoding the IgH and IgL chains are rearranged, proceeding through several stages from pro-B-cell to pre-B-cells, and finally immature-B cells. More in detail, VDJ recombination at the H chain locus results in the generation and surface expression of the pre-B-cell receptor (pre-BCR), formed by IgH and a surrogate IgL. This is replaced by a mature IgL following VJ recombination at the L chain locus, leading to the expression of a mature BCR. Following purging of self-reactive cells through negative selection, immature-B cells leave the BM as IgM^+ B cells to complete their development in the spleen, where they progress through transitional stages to generate mature follicular B cells or marginal-zone B cells co-expressing IgM and IgD. Following antigen recognition, antigen-specific B cells develop into either plasma cells or memory B cells [12, 13].

Similar to B cells, human NK cells develop from CLPs mainly in the BM, even though recent findings suggest that they can also develop in extramedullary sites such as secondary lymphoid tissues, liver, and others [14]. The irreversible fate commitment of CLPs to the NK cell lineage precursor (NKp) is defined by the expression of CD122 (IL-2Rβ) [15]. The acquisition of activating receptors such as CD314, CD335, CD337, and CD161 defines the immature NK cells (iNK) cells, while surface expression of CD56 (neural cell adhesion molecule) indicates the final transition of iNK to mature NK cells (mNK) [16] (Fig. 2.2).

A number of cellular defects are recognized as causing SCID, including impaired cell survival, defective response to cytokines, impaired assembly of the antigen receptor, and defective signaling [17]. These defects are associated with gene mutations that can exert their effects at different levels during lymphocyte development, accounting for different profiles of circulating lymphocytes in SCIDs.

In this chapter, we focus on the gene mutations associated with SCID and how they interfere with the maturation steps of the different cell lineages (Fig. 2.2).

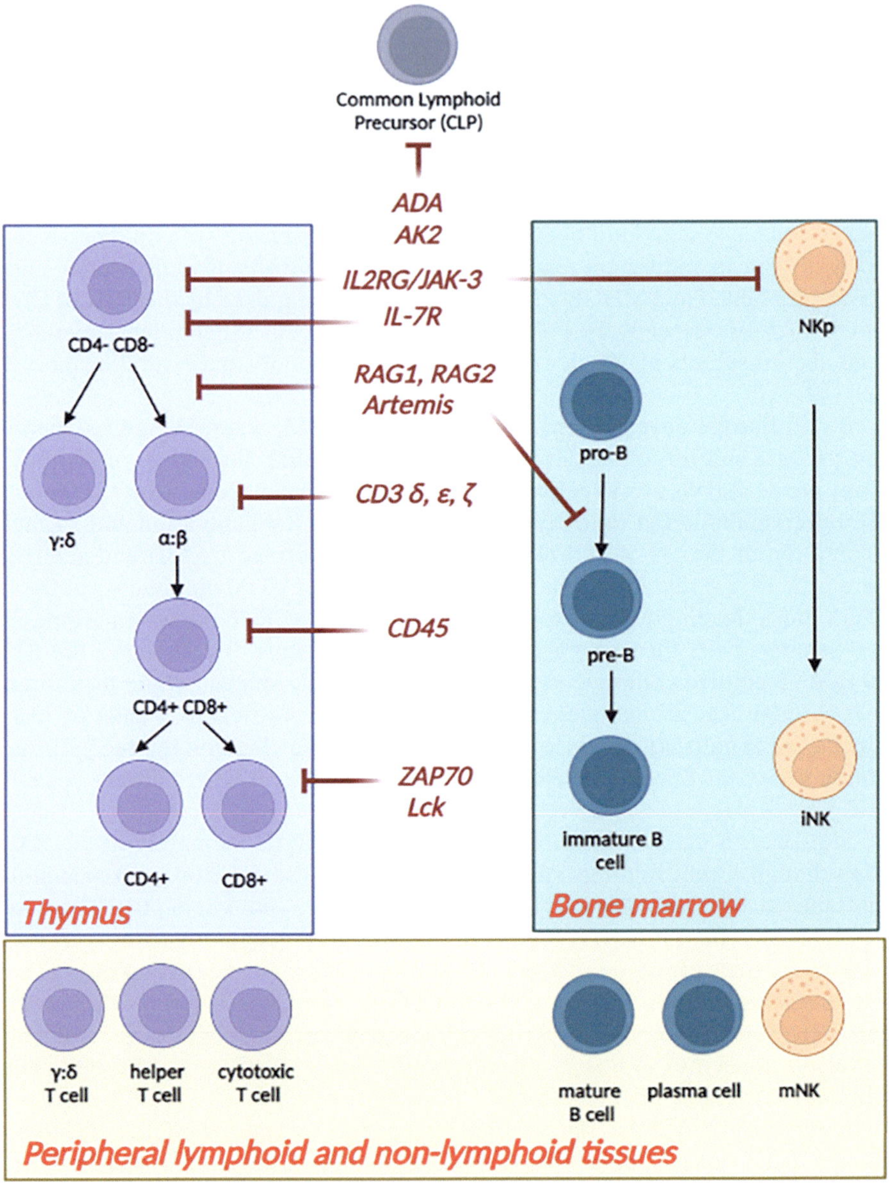

Fig. 2.2 Lymphoid development pathways and relative position of the gene defects underlying SCID

2.3 Genetic Defects in SCID and Their Impact on Lymphocyte Development

2.3.1 Early Impairment of the Common Lymphoid Progenitor

Some SCID-associated mutations act at the earliest stage of lymphocyte development, the CLP, thereby preventing the development of all cell types derived from this precursor, including T lymphocytes, B lymphocytes, and NK cells.

The most common defect associated with this phenotype is adenosine deaminase (ADA) deficiency. ADA deficiency is associated with mutations in the *ADA* gene, including missense, nonsense, and frameshift mutations, as well as splice-site mutations. ADA is a key enzyme in the purine metabolism pathway which irreversibly deaminates adenosine and deoxyadenosine to inosine and deoxyinosine, respectively. The disease is caused by a complete absence of ADA activity, which leads to the abnormal intracellular accumulation of adenosine, deoxyadenosine, and deoxyadenosine triphosphate that induce cell death by apoptosis. Of particular relevance for the clinical manifestations of SCID is the fact that CLPs are exquisitely sensitive to ADA deficiency-related apoptosis [18], resulting in the so-called $T^-B^-NK^-$ SCID profile, where the development of all the cell lineages is affected [19].

Another mutation resulting in a similar profile was observed in an autosomal recessive form of SCID, known as reticular dysgenesis (RD), characterized by an early arrest not only in CLP maturation but also in myeloid lineage differentiation. RD is associated with biallelic loss-of-function mutations in the *Adenylate Kinase 2* (*AK2*) gene, causing the loss of AK2 expression [20, 21]. AK2 is a phosphotransferase widely expressed in many tissues including all hematopoietic cells, where it mediates the phosphorylation of adenosine monophosphate (AMP) to adenosine diphosphate (ADP), the substrate for adenosine triphosphate (ATP) synthesis. Within the cell, AK2 localizes in the intermembrane space of mitochondria where it plays a key role in cellular and mitochondrial energy homeostasis and contributes to modulate the AMP-mediated response to stress signals. Deregulation of AK2 function has been involved in dysfunctional mitochondrial energy metabolism [22]. The mechanistic basis for the failure of myelopoiesis and lymphopoiesis in RD, however, remains unknown, although it may be caused by AMP accumulation which adversely affects ribonucleotide synthesis, a feature of AK2 deficiency.

2.3.2 Defective Signaling Through Cytokine Receptors

T-cell development and proliferation crucially depend upon cytokine signaling. Not surprisingly, mutations directly affecting receptors or other molecules involved in these signaling pathways have been associated to SCID.

Mutations in the *interleukin 2 receptor gamma chain* (*IL-2RG*) gene, encoding the common gamma chain (γc) of several cytokine receptors, are associated to X-linked SCID (X-SCID) [23, 24]. Approximately 250 mutations in *IL2RG* gene are known to cause SCID, including missense mutations, nonsense mutations, insertions, deletions, splice-site mutations, and mutations that affect RNA processing and translation [25, 26]. The lack of a functional *IL2RG* gene, hence, leads to the blockage of multiple cytokine pathways, whose receptors share the common γc, such as the IL-4, IL-7, IL-9, IL-15, and IL-21 receptors [27]. Early lymphoid progenitor cells, consequently, will be unable to respond to the signals triggered by these cytokines, which are essential for the normal development and function of T and NK cells. Hence, X-SCID is characterized by the so-called $T^-NK^-B^+$ profile, where T and NK cells are defective, while B cells are usually present; however, immunoglobulin production is severely reduced, if not absent [23, 28].

Mutations associated to the *Janus Kinase 3* (*JAK3*) gene are responsible for autosomal recessive SCID (AR-SCID). A large panel of *JAK3* mutations have been identified, which lead to a marked reduction or complete absence of JAK3 expression or function. Consistent with the signaling function of JAK3 in common γc-mediated cytokine signaling, *JAK3* mutations cause a phenotype indistinguishable from X-SCID, namely impaired T-cell development, signaling and survival at the early stages of T-cell maturation (DN thymocytes), as well as defective NK cell maturation [29–31].

Together with γc mutations, mutations in the gene encoding the IL-7 receptor (*IL7R*) have been implicated in SCID. Although only few patients with *IL7R* mutations have been studied, a number of mutations have been identified, the majority of which mapping to exon 4 [32]. Because of the key role of the IL7/IL7R axis in lymphocyte survival, proliferation and signaling, *IL7R* mutations, causing abnormal signal transduction, result in a profound and early block in T-cell differentiation while, surprisingly, B-cell development is entirely normal in *IL7R*-deficient patients [33], as opposed to mice where *IL7R* disruption severely impairs B-cell lymphopoiesis in the bone marrow [34].

2.3.3 Defective V(D)J Recombination

A major step in T- and B-lymphocyte differentiation is the somatic rearrangement of the antigen receptor, TCR and BCR, respectively. This process is initiated by the recombination-activating gene-1 (RAG-1) and RAG-2 proteins, which recognize the recombination signal sequences (RSS) flanking the V(D)J gene elements of the TCR and BCR chains and cleave the DNA at these specific sequences. Subsequently, the DNA double-strand break is resolved by the DNA cross-link repair 1C (DCLRE1C) protein, also known as Artemis, by the non-homologous end-joining (NHEJ) pathway, thereby permitting the juxtaposition of nonadjacent V(D)J gene segments [7].

Mutations in either *RAG1* or *RAG2*, as well as in *Artemis*, have been associated to SCID [35], with a variety of clinical and immunologic phenotypes. In patients with null *RAG* mutations, for example, complete failure of V(D)J recombination is associated with lack of circulating T and B lymphocytes, hence resulting in the $T^-B^-NK^+$ form of SCID. Hypomorphic *RAG* mutations that affect, but do not completely abolish, V(D)J recombination, are often associated with milder phenotypes, with residual presence of T and B cell, as observed in the Omenn syndrome [36–38].

Because RAG1/RAG2 and Artemis are required for the V(D)J rearrangement of the H chain and β chain locus in B and T cells, respectively, severe mutations of the respective genes block T-cell development prior to differentiation to single-positive thymocytes and B-cell development at the pro-B/pre-B transition. However, they are not required for NK cell development, and, consistently, mutations in these genes lead to a $T^-B^-NK^+$ SCID profile [39] (Fig. 2.1).

2.3.4 Defective CD3 Complex and Pre-TCR Signaling

During T-cell development the CD3 complex plays a key role in the transition of thymocytes from DN immature precursors to the $CD4^+CD8^+$ DP stage and finally to the mature SP T-cell [40]. In fact, intrathymic T lymphocyte differentiation requires appropriate signals from the pre-TCR and the three associated CD3 signal-transducing complexes, namely the CD3δε and CD3γε heterodimers and a disulfide-linked CD3ζζ. Selective deficiency of CD3 invariant chains CD3γ, δ, ε, and ζ can thus impacts on T-cell development, accounting however for only a small proportion of autosomal recessive SCID. The resulting phenotype is usually $T^-B^+NK^+$, but the clinical manifestations can vary depending on the deficient chain: patients with CD3δ, ε, and ζ deficiency have a typical severe SCID phenotype, while CD3γ deficiency results in a milder, non-fatal form of the disease [41–43].

Other types of SCID are caused to mutations in the genes encoding molecules involved in pre-TCR signaling. One example is the gene encoding CD45, a tyrosine phosphatase expressed on all leukocytes and required for efficient lymphocyte signaling. CD45-deficient mice are severely immunodeficient and have very few peripheral T lymphocytes. In the early 2000s, two different research groups identified two different clinical cases of SCID with mutations in the gene encoding CD45: the first patient characterized showed a large deletion at one *CD45* allele and a point mutation at the other allele [44], while the second patient had an homozygous 6-bp deletion associated with lack of CD45 surface expression [45]. In SCID patients, CD45 deficiency results mainly in T-cell dysfunction ($T^-B^+NK^+$ profile), even though serum immunoglobulin levels decreased with age in these patients despite normal B-lymphocyte numbers. Defects in other TCR signaling components have been implicated in SCID, such as mutations in the initiating kinases Lck and ZAP-70 [46]. ZAP-70 defects cause a characteristic deficiency of $CD8^+$ T lymphocytes, resulting in a $T^+(CD4^+CD8^-)B^+NK^+$ SCID [47], while Lck deficiency has been associated to CD4 lymphopenia [48]. Of note, as opposed to humans, ZAP-70-deficient mice have no mature $CD4^+$ or $CD8^+$ in the periphery as the result of a block in thymic development at the DP cells stage [49].

2.4 Conclusions and Future Perspectives

As described in this chapter, SCID includes a heterogeneous group of conditions, whose broad clinical and immunologic phenotype depends on the nature of the gene affected, and the specific mutations involved. Hence, knowledge of the different genetic and clinical forms of SCID is particularly relevant for a personalized approach to diagnosis and treatment.

Currently, the main treatment of SCID patients is hematopoietic stem cell transplantation (HSCT), and prognosis is generally good within the first few months of life and when an HLA (Human Leukocyte Antigen) matched donor is available [50]. More recently, in cases with graft versus host disease and graft rejection due to non-HLA identical donors, a gene therapy approach has been developed. It involves the isolation and *in vitro* correction of gene mutations in HSCTs from the patient, followed by transplantation of the engineered functional cells back into the patient himself. Numerous clinical trials based on gene therapy are ongoing, some of which seem to be particularly promising for children with X-SCID and ADA deficiency SCID [51]. Recently, an innovative gene therapy strategy has been developed by McAuley and colleagues, who used CRISPR-Cas9-based gene editing to correct a single base-pair mutation causing human CD3δ deficiency, with high efficiency and precision of genetic correction and low off-target effects [52]. An alternative therapeutical approach is represented by enzyme replacement therapy, useful for children and adults with ADA-SCID. In this type of treatment, ADA enzyme is periodically administered by intramuscular injection into patients resulting in a temporary relief. However, for long-term results also ADA-SCID patients have to resort to either HSCT or gene therapy [53].

Advances in diagnostic techniques and gene editing technologies, together with improved treatments, are required to increase survival and ameliorate the lifestyle of children with SCID.

References

1. Conley ME, Notarangelo LD, Etzioni A (1999) Diagnostic criteria for primary immunodeficiencies. Representing PAGID (Pan-American Group for Immunodeficiency) and ESID (European Society for Immunodeficiencies). Clin Immunol 93:190–197. https://doi.org/10.1006/clim.1999.4799
2. Gennery AR, Cant AJ (2001) Diagnosis of severe combined immunodeficiency. J Clin Pathol 54:191–195. https://doi.org/10.1136/jcp.54.3.191
3. McWilliams LM, Railey MD, Buckley RH (2015) Positive family history, infection, low absolute lymphocyte count (ALC), and absent thymic shadow: diagnostic clues for all molecular forms of severe combined immunodeficiency (SCID). J Allergy Clin Immunol Pract 3:585–591. https://doi.org/10.1016/j.jaip.2015.01.026
4. Fischer A, Le Deist F, Hacein-Bey-Abina S, André-Schmutz I, de Saint Basile G, de Villartay J et al (2005) Severe combined immunodeficiency. A model disease for molecular immunology and therapy. Immunol Rev 203:98–109. https://doi.org/10.1111/j.0105-2896.2005.00223.x
5. Aloj G, Giardino G, Valentino L, Maio F, Gallo V, Esposito T et al (2012) Severe combined immunodeficiences: new and old scenarios. Int Rev Immunol 31:43–65. https://doi.org/10.3109/08830185.2011.644607
6. Hesslein DG, Schatz DG (2001) Factors and forces controlling V(D)J recombination. Adv Immunol 78:169–232. https://doi.org/10.1016/s0065-2776(01)78004-2
7. Bassing CH, Swat W, Alt FW (2002) The mechanism and regulation of chromosomal V(D)J recombination. Cell 109(Suppl):S45–S55. https://doi.org/10.1016/s0092-8674(02)00675-x
8. Zúñiga-Pflücker JC (2004) T-cell development made simple. Nat Rev Immunol 4:67–72. https://doi.org/10.1038/nri1257
9. Sallusto F, Geginat J, Lanzavecchia A (2004) Central memory and effector memory T cell subsets: function, generation, and maintenance. Annu Rev Immunol 22:745–763. https://doi.org/10.1146/annurev.immunol.22.012703.104702

10. Kaech SM, Cui W (2012) Transcriptional control of effector and memory CD8+ T cell differentiation. Nat Rev Immunol 12:749–761. https://doi.org/10.1038/nri3307
11. Ruterbusch M, Pruner KB, Shehata L, Pepper M (2020) In vivo CD4+ T cell differentiation and function: revisiting the Th1/Th2 paradigm. Annu Rev Immunol 38:705–725. https://doi.org/10.1146/annurev-immunol-103019-085803
12. Melchers F (2015) Checkpoints that control B cell development. J Clin Invest 125:2203–2210. https://doi.org/10.1172/JCI78083
13. Wang Y, Liu J, Burrows PD, Wang J (2020) B cell development and maturation. Adv Exp Med Biol 1254:1–22. https://doi.org/10.1007/978-981-15-3532-1_1
14. Scoville SD, Freud AG, Caligiuri MA (2017) Modeling human natural killer cell development in the era of innate lymphoid cells. Front Immunol 8:360. https://doi.org/10.3389/fimmu.2017.00360
15. Yu J, Freud AG, Caligiuri MA (2013) Location and cellular stages of natural killer cell development. Trends Immunol 34:573–582. https://doi.org/10.1016/j.it.2013.07.005
16. Di Vito C, Mikulak J, Mavilio D (2019) On the way to become a natural killer cell. Front Immunol 10:1812. https://doi.org/10.3389/fimmu.2019.01812
17. Buckley RH (2004) Molecular defects in human severe combined immunodeficiency and approaches to immune reconstitution. Annu Rev Immunol 22:625–655. https://doi.org/10.1146/annurev.immunol.22.012703.104614
18. Hershfield MS (2003) Genotype is an important determinant of phenotype in adenosine deaminase deficiency. Curr Opin Immunol 15:571–577. https://doi.org/10.1016/s0952-7915(03)00104-3
19. Ozdemir O (2006) Severe combined immune deficiency in an adenosine deaminase-deficient patient. Allergy Asthma Proc 27:172–174
20. Lagresle-Peyrou C, Six EM, Picard C, Rieux-Laucat F, Michel V, Ditadi A et al (2009) Human adenylate kinase 2 deficiency causes a profound hematopoietic defect associated with sensorineural deafness. Nat Genet 41:106–111. https://doi.org/10.1038/ng.278
21. Pannicke U, Hönig M, Hess I, Friesen C, Holzmann K, Rump E et al (2009) Reticular dysgenesis (aleukocytosis) is caused by mutations in the gene encoding mitochondrial adenylate kinase 2. Nat Genet 41:101–105. https://doi.org/10.1038/ng.265
22. Dzeja P, Terzic A (2009) Adenylate kinase and AMP signaling networks: metabolic monitoring, signal communication and body energy sensing. Int J Mol Sci 10:1729–1772. https://doi.org/10.3390/ijms10041729
23. Noguchi M, Yi H, Rosenblatt HM, Filipovich AH, Adelstein S, Modi WS et al (1993) Interleukin-2 receptor gamma chain mutation results in X-linked severe combined immunodeficiency in humans. Cell 73:147–157. https://doi.org/10.1016/0092-8674(93)90167-o
24. Leonard WJ (2001) Cytokines and immunodeficiency diseases. Nat Rev Immunol 1:200–208. https://doi.org/10.1038/35105066
25. DiSanto JP, Rieux-Laucat F, Dautry-Varsat A, Fischer A, de Saint Basile G (1994) Defective human interleukin 2 receptor gamma chain in an atypical X chromosome-linked severe combined immunodeficiency with peripheral T cells. Proc Natl Acad Sci USA 91:9466–9470. https://doi.org/10.1073/pnas.91.20.9466
26. Puck J, Pepper A, Henthorn P, Candotti F, Isakov J, Whitwam T et al (1997) Mutation analysis of IL2RG in human X-linked severe combined immunodeficiency. Blood 89:1968–1977
27. Matthews DJ, Clark PA, Herbert J, Morgan G, Armitage RJ, Kinnon C et al (1995) Function of the interleukin-2 (IL-2) receptor gamma-chain in biologic responses of X-linked severe combined immunodeficient B cells to IL-2, IL-4, IL-13, and IL-15. Blood 85:38–42
28. Leonard WJ, Shores EW, Love PE (1995) Role of the common cytokine receptor gamma chain in cytokine signaling and lymphoid development. Immunol Rev 148:97–114. https://doi.org/10.1111/j.1600-065x.1995.tb00095.x
29. Macchi P, Villa A, Giliani S, Sacco MG, Frattini A, Porta F et al (1995) Mutations of Jak-3 gene in patients with autosomal severe combined immune deficiency (SCID). Nature 377:65–68. https://doi.org/10.1038/377065a0

30. Park SY, Saijo K, Takahashi T, Osawa M, Arase H, Hirayama N et al (1995) Developmental defects of lymphoid cells in Jak3 kinase-deficient mice. Immunity 3:771–782. https://doi.org/10.1016/1074-7613(95)90066-7
31. Russell SM, Tayebi N, Nakajima H, Riedy MC, Roberts JL, Aman MJ et al (1995) Mutation of Jak3 in a patient with SCID: essential role of Jak3 in lymphoid development. Science 270:797–800. https://doi.org/10.1126/science.270.5237.797
32. Hamosh A, Scott AF, Amberger J, Bocchini C, Valle D, McKusick VA (2002) Online Mendelian Inheritance in Man (OMIM), a knowledgebase of human genes and genetic disorders. Nucleic Acids Res 30:52–55. https://doi.org/10.1093/nar/30.1.52
33. Puel A, Ziegler S, Buckley R, Leonard W (1998) Defective IL7R expression in T(−) B(+)NK(+) severe combined immunodeficiency. Nat Genet 20:394–397. https://doi.org/10.1038/3877
34. Peschon JJ, Morrissey PJ, Grabstein KH, Ramsdell FJ, Maraskovsky E, Gliniak BC et al (1994) Early lymphocyte expansion is severely impaired in interleukin 7 receptor-deficient mice. J Exp Med 180:1955–1960. https://doi.org/10.1084/jem.180.5.1955
35. Moshous D, Callebaut I, de Chasseval R, Corneo B, Cavazzana-Calvo M, Le Deist F et al (2001) Artemis, a novel DNA double-strand break repair/V(D)J recombination protein is mutated in human severe combined immune deficiency with increased radiosensitivity (RS-SCID). Cell 105:177–186. https://doi.org/10.1016/s0092-8674(01)00309-9
36. Villa A, Santagata S, Bozzi F, Giliani S, Frattini A, Imberti L et al (1998) Partial V(D)J recombination activity leads to Omenn syndrome. Cell 93:885–896. https://doi.org/10.1016/s0092-8674(00)81448-8
37. Abolhassani H, Wang N, Aghamohammadi A, Rezaei N, Lee YN, Frugoni F et al (2014) A hypomorphic recombination-activating gene 1 (RAG1) mutation resulting in a phenotype resembling common variable immunodeficiency. J Allergy Clin Immunol 134:1375–1380. https://doi.org/10.1016/j.jaci.2014.04.042
38. Giblin W, Chatterji M, Westfield G, Masud T, Theisen B, Cheng H et al (2009) Leaky severe combined immunodeficiency and aberrant DNA rearrangements due to a hypomorphic RAG1 mutation. Blood 113:2965–2975. https://doi.org/10.1182/blood-2008-07-165167
39. Gennery A (2019) Recent advances in understanding RAG deficiencies. F1000Res 8:F1000 Faculty Rev-148. https://doi.org/10.12688/f1000research.17056.1
40. von Boehmer H, Fehling HJ (1997) Structure and function of the pre-T cell receptor. Annu Rev Immunol 15:433–452. https://doi.org/10.1146/annurev.immunol.15.1.433
41. Dadi HK, Simon AJ, Roifman CM (2003) Effect of CD3δ deficiency on maturation of α/β and γ/δ T-cell lineages in severe combined immunodeficiency. N Engl J Med 349:1821–1828. https://doi.org/10.1056/NEJMoa031178
42. de Saint Basile G, Geissmann F, Flori E, Uring-Lambert B, Soudais C, Cavazzana-Calvo M et al (2004) Severe combined immunodeficiency caused by deficiency in either the δ or the ε subunit of CD3. J Clin Invest 114:1512–1517. https://doi.org/10.1172/JCI22588
43. Tokgoz H, Caliskan U, Keles S, Reisli I, Guiu IS, Morgan NV (2013) Variable presentation of primary immune deficiency: two cases with CD3 gamma deficiency presenting with only autoimmunity. Pediatr Allergy Immunol 24:257–262. https://doi.org/10.1111/pai.12063
44. Kung C, Pingel JT, Heikinheimo M, Klemola T, Varkila K, Yoo LI et al (2000) Mutations in the tyrosine phosphatase CD45 gene in a child with severe combined immunodeficiency disease. Nat Med 6:343–345. https://doi.org/10.1038/73208
45. Tchilian EZ, Wallace DL, Wells RS, Flower DR, Morgan G, Beverley PC (2001) A deletion in the gene encoding the CD45 antigen in a patient with SCID. J Immunol 166:1308–1313. https://doi.org/10.4049/jimmunol.166.2.1308
46. Cossu F (2010) Genetics of SCID. Ital J Pediatr 36:76. https://doi.org/10.1186/1824-7288-36-76
47. Turul T, Tezcan I, Artac H, de Bruin-Versteeg S, Barendregt BH, Reisli I et al (2009) Clinical heterogeneity can hamper the diagnosis of patients with ZAP70 deficiency. Eur J Pediatr 168:87–93. https://doi.org/10.1007/s00431-008-0718-x

48. Hubert P, Bergeron F, Ferreira V, Seligmann M, Oksenhendler E, Debre P et al (2000) Defective p56Lck activity in T cells from an adult patient with idiopathic CD4+ lymphocytopenia. Int Immunol 12:449–457. https://doi.org/10.1093/intimm/12.4.449
49. Negishi I, Motoyama N, Nakayama K, Nakayama K, Senju S, Hatakeyama S et al (1995) Essential role for ZAP-70 in both positive and negative selection of thymocytes. Nature 376:435–438. https://doi.org/10.1038/376435a0
50. Castagnoli R, Delmonte OM, Calzoni E, Notarangelo LD (2019) Hematopoietic stem cell transplantation in primary immunodeficiency diseases: current status and future perspectives. Front Pediatr 7:295. https://doi.org/10.3389/fped.2019.00295
51. Fischer A, Hacein-Bey-Abina S (2020) Gene therapy for severe combined immunodeficiencies and beyond. J Exp Med 217:e20190607. https://doi.org/10.1084/jem.20190607
52. McAuley GE, Yiu G, Chang PC, Newby GA, Campo-Fernandez B, Fitz-Gibbon ST et al (2023) Human T cell generation is restored in CD3δ severe combined immunodeficiency through adenine base editing. Cell 186:1398–1416.e23. https://doi.org/10.1016/j.cell.2023.02.027
53. Secord E, Hartog NL (2022) Review of treatment for adenosine deaminase deficiency (ADA) severe combined immunodeficiency (SCID). Ther Clin Risk Manag 18:939–944. https://doi.org/10.2147/TCRM.S350762

Bioinformatics in Primary Immunodeficiencies: Towards a "Computational Immunology" Era

3

Josefina del Pilar Martínez Vásquez
and Alexios-Fotios Mentis

Abbreviations

AUC	Area under the curve
BAM	Binary Alignment Map
BCRs	B-cell receptors
BN	Bayesian network
CBTOPE	Conformational B-cell epitope prediction
CDS	Clinical decision support
CID	Combined immunodeficiency
CNVs	Copy number variations
CTLA-4	Cytotoxic T-lymphocyte associated protein 4
CVID	Common variable immunodeficiency
DDR	Deoxynucleotide triphosphates
DEGs	Differentially expressed genes
DKMS	Deutsche Knochenmarkspenderdatei (German Bone Marrow Donor Center)
EHR	Electronic Health Records
EPIMHC	Epitope prediction using integrated methods for HLA binding prediction and comparison
ESP	Exome sequencing project
FACS	Fluorescence-activated cell sorting
GC-MS	Gas chromatography coupled with mass spectrometry

J. d. P. Martínez Vásquez
Area of Basic and Environmental Sciences, Instituto Tecnológico de Santo Domingo, Santo Domingo, Dominican Republic

A.-F. Mentis (✉)
BGI-Shenzhen, Shenzhen, Guangdong, China
e-mail: amentis1@alumni.jh.edu

M. M. D'Elios (ed.), *Severe Combined Immunodeficiency*, Rare Diseases of the Immune System, https://doi.org/10.1007/978-3-031-78864-2_3

GDPR	General Data Protection Regulation
gnomAD	Genome Aggregation Database
GRNs	Gene regulation networks
HGVP	Human Genetic Variation Database
HLA	Human leukocyte antigen
HMP DACC	Human Microbiome Project Data Analysis and Coordination Center
HPO	Human Phenotype Ontology
IEDB	Immune Epitope Database
IL-2	Interleukin-2
IMG/M	Integrated Microbial Genomes with Microbiome Samples
LC-MS	Liquid chromatography coupled with mass spectrometry
LPS	Lipopolysaccharide
LR	Logistic regression
LRBA	Lipopolysaccharide-responsive and Beige-like anchor protein
MAFs	Minor allele frequencies
MetaPhlAn	Metagenomic Phylogenetic Analysis
MG-RAST	Metagenomics Rapid Annotation using Subsystem Technology
MHC	Major histocompatibility complex
MM	Motif matrices
mNGS	Metagenomic shotgun next-generation sequencing
NCBI	National Center for Biotechnology Information
NetCDF	Network Common Data Form
NGS	Next-generation sequencing
NLP	Natural language processing
OMIM	Online Mendelian Inheritance in Man
PATRIC	Pathosystems Resource Integration Center
PCR	Polymerase chain reaction
PI3Kδ	Phosphatidylinositol 3 kinase delta
PID	Primary immunodeficiency
PIDs	Primary immunodeficiencies
PIK3R1	Phosphoinositide-3-kinase regulatory subunit 1
PROVEAN	Protein Variation Effect Analyzer
PyMOL	Python molecular viewer
QAMs	Quantitative affinity matrices
QC	Quality control
RCSB	Research Collaboratory for Structural Bioinformatics
RT	Retention time
SAM	Sequence Alignment Map
sCD14	Soluble cluster of differentiation 14
sCD25	Soluble cluster of differentiation 25
SCID	Severe combined immunodeficiency
SIFT	Sorting Intolerant From Tolerant
SNVs	Single nucleotide variants
SVM	Support vector machine
SVMtrip	Support vector machine based on tri-peptide composition

SVs	Structural variations
TAP	Transporters associated with antigen processing
TNF-α	Tumor necrosis factor alpha
UMIs	Unique molecular identifiers
UniProt	Universal protein resource
VCF	Variant call format
VMD	Visual molecular dynamics
WES	Whole exome sequencing
WGS	Whole genome sequencing
ZKRD	Zentrales Knochenmarkspender-Register Deutschland (Central Bone Marrow Donor Registry Germany)

3.1 Introduction to Computational Immunology

The immune system is composed of a set of proteins, cells, and signaling pathways that protect the body from viruses, infections, autoimmune responses, cancerous cells, and inflammatory disorders [1]. Dysregulation of the immune system leads to difficult-to-diagnose disorders, including primary immunodeficiencies (PID), characterized by defective immune responses, which, in turn, increase susceptibility to infections, autoimmune reactions, and inflammation [2]. Given its nodal role in human (patho)physiology, understanding the immune system is essential for comprehending cellular defense mechanisms, developing novel treatments, and improving general health status. The field of "Computational immunology" has emerged because of advances in computational biology and multi-omics approaches, which use high-throughput genomic and bioinformatics tools to turn immunology datasets into computationally accessible information [3]. This chapter will aim to cover next-generation sequencing techniques, structural bioinformatics, data integration, bioinformatics for drug discovery, and artificial intelligence in the diagnosis of primary immunodeficiencies, as well as to highlight future directions in computational immunology.

3.2 Genomic Approaches in Immunodeficiency Research: A Structured Approach Towards Whole Genome Sequencing

Over 360 genes have already been linked to immunodeficiencies [4]. Prognosis, treatment planning, and genetic counseling all depend on an accurate diagnosis. Nevertheless, achieving a precise molecular diagnosis is challenging because of the phenotypic and genotypic diversity, which produces aberrant presentations and symptoms that tend to overlap. Genomics provides important insights by analyzing an organism's whole genome, and it has transformed how disease-related gene panels are assessed in terms of their diagnostic potential, thus representing an increasingly appreciated solution to diagnostic challenges [5].

Understanding genetic variations is critical to diagnose primary immunodeficiencies. To achieve precise genetic profiling, high-throughput next-generation sequencing methodologies must be chosen, considering the scalability for effective resource allocation, optimal extraction of genetic information, cost reduction, and simplified data management [6]. In this context, both standard and next-generation sequencing approaches for diagnosing primary immunodeficiency are presented below, along with case examples illustrating the efficacy and scalability of these genomics-driven approaches.

3.2.1 A Structured Approach Towards DNA Sequencing and Its Use in the Diagnosis of Primary Immunodeficiencies

3.2.1.1 Sanger Sequencing

Sanger sequencing uses deoxynucleotide triphosphates (dNTPs) and a DNA polymerase to incorporate nucleotides. Chain extension stops when fluorophore-labeled fluorescently labeled dideoxynucleotides triphosphates (ddNTPs) bind, thus creating distinct fluorophore-labeled fragments. Capillary gel electrophoresis separates fragments by molecular mass, and a charge-coupled device quantifies fluorescence, generating a chromatogram [7]. Sanger sequencing is nowadays a reliable diagnostic method, and it is cost-effective for several mutations, especially those with a familial history of known pathogenic variants and those due to substitutions (see Box 3.1). Now representing the "gold standard," it confirms next-generation sequencing results for targeted gene panels and whole exome sequencing. Despite its ability to cover any genomic region, Sanger sequencing's higher cost makes gene-specific assays more commonly used in clinical practice. Due to the high genetic diversity in PID symptoms, single-gene testing is impractical, as notably seen in primary antibody deficiency, where variations may occur in any of the around 40 genes discovered so far. This lack of efficiency and high expense have prompted the preference for high-throughput methods including gene panels, exome sequencing, or whole genome sequencing in PID investigations, avoiding labor-intensive and non-automated Sanger sequencing [8–10].

Box 3.1 Case Study 1: Single Gene Test—Autoimmunity and Recurring Infections Caused by a *STAT1* Gain-of-Function Mutation

A 3-year-old girl presents recurrent *Candida albicans* and bacterial infections, autoimmune manifestations, and a lupus-like syndrome but with normal serum immunoglobulins and lymphocyte counts. A heterozygous mutation (P293L) leading to a gain-of-function in the STAT1 coiled-coil domain was discovered by Sanger sequencing [11]. This case exemplifies the efficacy of single-gene testing using the Sanger algorithm for well-characterized disorders: *STAT1* Gain-of-Function mutation testing has gained recent attention in individuals experiencing persistent candidiasis and recurring infections, as these mutations account for almost half of the reported cases of chronic mucocutaneous candidiasis (CMC) [12]. Focusing on the STAT1 gene associated, Sanger sequencing provided a precise and cost-effective method. In cases where broader genetic exploration is needed, methods like gene panels, whole exome sequencing (WES), and whole genome sequencing (WGS) can be employed.

3.2.1.2 Next-Generation Sequencing

Next-Generation Sequencing (NGS) refers to the massive parallelization of DNA fragment sequencing. DNA is isolated from the tissue sample, and its quality, yield, and concentration are assessed to ensure suitability for sequencing. DNA libraries are prepared by fragmenting the input DNA, adding short adapter sequences, performing size selection, and applying PCR-based amplification. Indexing assigns unique codes to samples, thus cutting per-sample sequencing costs and simplifying distribution over numerous lanes. Indexes can be incorporated into adapters or added during PCR enrichment [13] (see Fig. 3.1). In addition, Table 3.1 offers an overview of current DNA sequencing technology, highlighting several techniques via key platforms.

Box 3.2 Fasta File Creation

- **Binary Base Call (BCL)**: Initial NGS data, which contain the fluorescent signals for each called base on a sequencing chip. Software such as TagGD, DigestFlow, or Illumina's Bcl2fastq are applied. Conversion software demultiplexes BCL files into FASTA or FASTQ formats. This process transforms base calls and Q-scores in BCL files into DNA sequences and quality strings saved in structured plain-text files [15].
- **FASTA files**: They provide sequence descriptions and nucleotide sequences with single-letter codes, starting with a ">" description line. Keeping lines under 80 characters is advisable for clarity [21].
- **FASTQ**: The standard format for storing NGS data is called FASTQ. It contains a Sequence ID, raw nucleotide sequence, separator, and a line denoting nucleotide quality that makes up its four lines [21].

Genome Alignment

Genome alignment most frequently utilizes the GRCh38 or hg38 human reference genome to identify functional, structural, and evolutionary connections among sequences [6]. Tools such as BWA [22], Bowtie [23], Kart [24], Novoalign [25], and Minimap2 [26] are commonly used; however, their limitation lies in every platform's specificity for all these tools [9].

Sequence alignment results go into Sequence Alignment Map (SAM) or its compressed binary form, Binary Alignment Map (BAM). BAM offers several

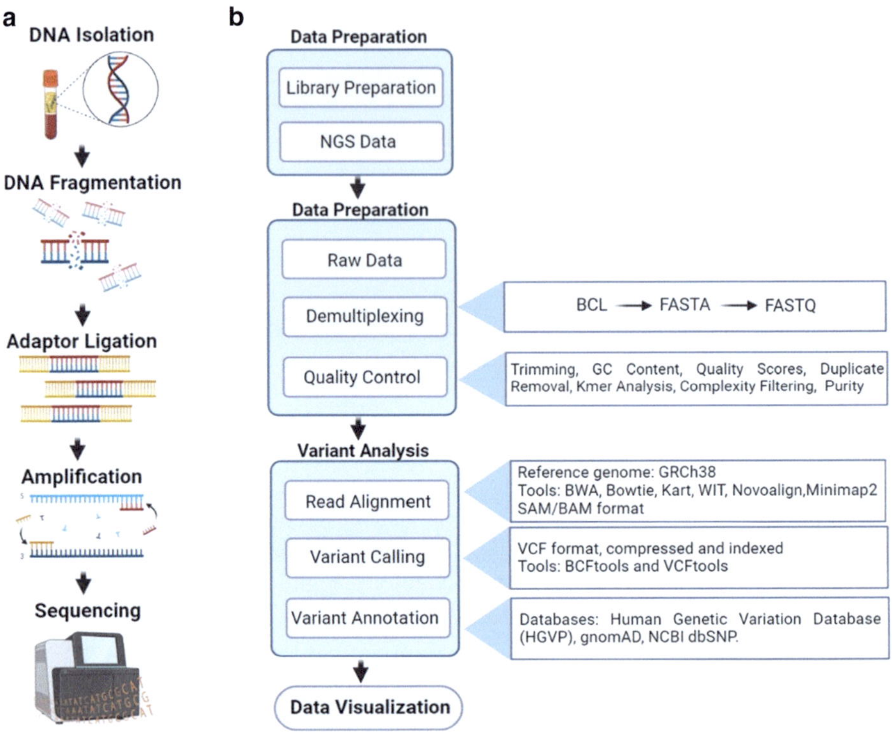

Fig. 3.1 Next-generation sequencing workflow. (**a**) NGS wet laboratory workflow begins with DNA isolation from a tissue sample, assessing quality, yield, and concentration for sequencing suitability. The process includes library preparation with DNA fragmentation, adapter addition, size selection, and PCR amplification. Notably, indexing is introduced, assigning unique codes to samples, reducing per-sample costs, and facilitating efficient distribution across multiple sequencing lanes. Indexes can be incorporated into adapters or introduced during PCR enrichment, enhancing overall NGS workflow efficiency. (**b**) Data Analysis: raw data acquisition, progresses through demultiplexing and quality control and details the BCL to FASTQ conversion, including trimming, GC content analysis, and duplicate removal. The variant analysis section covers read alignment (GRCh38, BWA, Bowtie, Kart, WIT, Novoalign, Minimap2), variant calling (VCF format, BCFtools, VCftools), and annotation using HGVP, gnomAD, and NCBI dbSNP databases (for the steps of creating a FASTA/FASTQ file, see Box 3.2). This succinct overview captures the essential components of the sequencing and variant analysis workflow. (Adapted from: Ona [14] and Lalrinmawii et al. [15])

advantages, i.e., (a) It is compressed for efficient storage and transfer; (b) It consolidates all alignment details into a single row for straightforward processing; (c) It is indexed to facilitate rapid region-specific access; and (d) It supports visualization in tools such as the Integrative Genomics Viewer and the University of California Santa Cruz (UCSC) Genome Browser for manually evaluating genetic variations [27].

Before calling variants, SAM/BAM file quality control checks sequencing metrics, coverage depth, duplicate read percentage, and sample contamination. The

Table 3.1 Overview of DNA sequencing technologies

Technology	Examples	Description
Sanger sequencing	ABI 3730xl, Applied Biosystems	ddNTPs cause DNA synthesis to stop, resulting in DNA fragments of different lengths. Electrophoresis is used to separate the fragments, and then the sequence is established [8]
Sequencing by synthesis	Illumina HiSeq, NovaSeq, Illumina (Solexa) sequencing	Adapters are introduced following the DNA fragmentation. After the fragments have been attached to a flow cell, synthesis-based sequencing takes place. A specific fluorescent signal is emitted for each base, allowing its identification [16]
Ion torrent sequencing	Ion Torrent PGM, Ion GeneStudio	During DNA elongation, as nucleotides are incorporated, hydrogen ions are released, thus changing the pH of the solution. An analysis of pH variations reveals the sequence [17]
Single-molecule real-time sequencing	PacBio Sequel, Sequel II	DNA is synthesized by a polymerase, and light released during nucleotide incorporation is captured by a zero-mode waveguide. This produces lengthy readings with high accuracy [18]
Oxford nanopore sequencing	MinION, GridION, PromethION	Nucleotide sequences are identified in real-time by DNA flowing through protein nanopores, which causes changes in electrical current [19]
454 Pyrosequencing	454 GS FLX Titanium	Following the insertion of an adapter and DNA fragmentation, the fragments are attached to beads, and they release pyrophosphate when nucleotides are incorporated, thus enabling base identification [20]

depth of coverage, which is commonly identified as the average number of unduplicated reads in the target area, is critical for variant finding confidence [28]. Picard Tools [29] and Qualimap [30] are two common tools for quality control procedures, with MultiQC [31] combining results from numerous bioinformatic software and studies into an individual report.

Variant Annotation and Identification

Somatic variants are examined in the results of BAM alignment, and genetic differences are identified through variant calling, which is performed by algorithms called variant callers. For effective management, the resultant call set is usually provided in variant call format (VCF), a compressed and indexed file. For modifying VCF files in genomic data analysis, BCFtools and VCFtools are frequently utilized [32]. To detect known variants, the call set is frequently annotated with population data from databases such as the Human Genetic Variation Database (HGVP) [33], gnomAD [34], and NCBI dbSNP [35].

Using annotation tools such as Ensembl VEP [36], ANNOVAR [37], and GATK Funcotator [38], variant analysis is completed by identifying SNVs, indels, CNVs, and SVs and by assessing their biological significance, gene impact, splicing effects, and pathogenicity. The next step is to apply filtering, such as population filtering for germline variations to eliminate artifacts and lower false positives. Sanger sequencing and other orthogonal techniques can also confirm a subset of variations [39]. Through manual examination, genuine and spurious deletions in CNVs and SVs are distinguished using methods such as Samplot and Samplot-ML [40].

Incorporating Insights on Bioinformatics Algorithms for Novel Variant Classification

Bioinformatics algorithms for novel variant classification analyze large-scale genomic data, annotating variants by identifying their location, functional consequences, and potential impact on protein structure or function, and comparing variants with population databases for frequency assessment to predict pathogenicity [41]. Fang et al.'s VIPPID is a specialized SNV pathogenicity prediction tool for PIDs. It addresses the challenge of distinguishing pathogenic from non-pathogenic variants by employing gene-specific models for the most common PID genes. VIPPID outperforms non-specific tools with an area under the curve (AUC) equal to 0.91 [42]. On the other hand, the groundbreaking concept of the "human gene connectome," which has been introduced by Itan and Casanova, functions as a biological Global Positioning System (GPS). This system ranks genes based on their similarity to known PID genes, generating an initial list of 3110 potential PID-causing genes. This method offers a systematic approach for researchers and clinicians, and it promises early diagnosis, treatment, and genetic counseling in PID, thus advancing our understanding and patient care significantly [43].

References to Omim, ClinVar, and Other Pertinent Databases

Human genomic databases, which are targeted towards specific genes, populations, or ethnic groups, facilitate DNA-level diagnosis by associating different genomic variants with unique phenotypic patterns and clinical characteristics. These libraries effectively arrange information and variations, providing useful tools for molecular diagnosis and aiding researchers and physicians in their endeavors [44].

Variant databases such as GnomAD [34], ESP [34], and ExAC [45] are crucial for determining Minor Allele Frequencies (MAFs) in diverse populations, aiding in distinguishing disease and non-disease states. Excessive MAFs indicate benignity, while their absence or lower carrier frequency provides moderate evidence for pathogenicity. The NCBI, using tools like the Variation Viewer [46], allows simultaneous MAF review across ESP [34], ExAC [45], and the One Thousand Genomes Project [47]. Table 3.2 compiles essential genomic databases and tools for thorough variant analysis.

3.2.1.3 Gene Panel Sequencing

Gene panels represent carefully curated collections of genes, ranging from a few to over a thousand genes, which use NGS and probes to identify specific coding areas [57]. This method ensures high accuracy, sensitivity, and efficient analysis, collectively accelerating PID diagnosis. It consists of a more cost-effective approach than whole exome sequencing (WES) and whole genome sequencing (WGS) in cases where the underlying causing gene is suspected, and it is frequently used in clinical diagnostics for rare diseases. It also yields faster results than Sanger sequencing,

Table 3.2 Overview of genomic databases and tools for variant analysis

Category	Examples	Purpose and features
Variant databases	• GnomAD [34] • ESP [34] • ExAC [45] • NCBI Variation Viewer [46] • 1000 Genomes Project [47]	Aid in distinguishing disease and non-disease states by determining Minor Allele Frequencies (MAFs) in diverse populations. A high MAF suggests benignity, while absence or low frequency provides moderate evidence for pathogenicity [48]
Disease-specific databases	• ClinVar [49]	Include information on diseases, syndromes, and other medical disorders, symptoms, signs, risk factors, treatment plans, and results from relevant research studies [50]
Functional validation	• OMIM [51] • HPO [52]	Establish the biological and functional importance of polymorphisms by linking them to phenotypes. This approach allows the confirmation of genetic variants' significance and their impact on human disorders [53]
Plausibility assessment	• UniProt [54] • InterPro [55] • Swiss-Model [56]	Contributes to assessing the plausibility of PIDD variants. It includes protein structure impact and tissue-specific gene expression analysis [44]

and it provides deeper sequencing capabilities (for a case study on the value of gene panels, see Box 3.3). Although gene panel sequencing cannot identify new causally implicated genes or structural changes (such as copy number variations), it provides a high-read depth at a low cost, which is especially advantageous for health systems in resource-poor settings. However, because full coverage is limited, a cautious interpretation of negative findings is required [58]. Moreover, gene panels have limitations in detecting variants which are not covered by the panel, such as mutations in non-coding areas, and variants in newly identified genes that are not yet linked to human disorders [59].

Box 3.3 Case Study 2: Gene Panel Testing—X-Linked *SASH3* Deficiency Presenting as a Common Variable Immunodeficiency

A 43-year-old man presented with persistent upper tract infections, low IgG and low IgM, and a history of severe varicella-zoster virus, minor warts, and bilateral pneumonia due to influenza, all of which suggested a possible case of common variable immunodeficiency (CVID). The patient's history of severe viral infections led to a request for a second medical opinion after the initial diagnosis of CVID. A hemizygous variation (c.505C>T/p.Gln169*) in the *SASH3* gene was discovered by employing a Next-Generation Sequencing (NGS) gene panel comprising 427 genes linked to Inborn Errors of Immunity [60]. The gene panel found a pathogenic variant in the *SASH3* gene, suggesting a highly likely Combined Immunodeficiency (CID) diagnosis. The patient's recurring infections suggested a high possibility of inborn defects of immunity-associated genes, which is why gene panel testing was chosen. This focused method proved cheaper and more useful than Sanger sequencing, as the latter can only assess each gene separately. The clinical presentation indicated a well-defined genetic disease, thus WES and WGS approaches were not pursued.

3.2.1.4 Whole Exome Sequencing

Whole Exome Sequencing (WES) is a sophisticated method that focuses on sequencing an individual's protein-coding genes ("exome"). It provides a more thorough examination of exonic regions compared to gene panels, allowing the identification of a wider variety of genetic variations, including novel structural variations. Despite potential trade-offs in read depth, WES is valuable for pinpointing specific genetic variations related to immune system deficits and for customizing treatment options. WES offers several advantages, including simultaneous testing of a broad spectrum of genes with high accuracy, faster results, and cost-effectiveness compared to whole genome sequencing (WGS) [61].

WES is potent in identifying genetic causes for rare diseases, especially in the so-called "trio analysis," which consists of sequencing both parents and the proband (for a successful case study where WES was applied, see Box 3.4). Nonetheless, challenges in WES include interpreting numerous variants, generating variants of undetermined significance (VUS), an increased risk of incidental findings, and limitations in detecting mosaicism or variants in non-coding regions. Technical challenges in short-read sequencing may hinder analysis, and despite broader genomic coverage, WES data analysis is more time-consuming than gene panel analysis, thus affecting turnaround time in clinical reporting [62]. While WES demonstrates a diagnostic yield of around 25% in the sum of genomic-driven diagnostic evaluations, it may overlook clinically relevant variants lying in non-protein coding regions. In cases where individuals remain undiagnosed after WES, additional genomic testing, such as WGS, should be considered to enhance the chances of identifying relevant variants [63].

Box 3.4 Case Study 3: Whole Exome Sequencing (WES)—Strong Combined Immunodeficiency Syndrome (SCID)

A 5-month-old girl presented with liver and spleen enlargement, ulcers in the mouth, depletion of T cells, recurrent fever, and frequent bacterial as well as viral infections. WES was employed to identify the genetic etiology of these symptoms. The *IL7R* gene included a 268 kb deletion and a splicing variation, (c.221 + 1G > A). This is the first report of an *IL7R* gene deletion and harmful splicing variation in a SCID patient [64]. WES is a thorough and effective method for determining the genetic basis of complex disorders such as SCID, thus allowing for early and precise diagnosis. Due to the genetic variability of SCID, Sanger sequencing and gene panels might miss rare mutations, while Whole Genome Sequencing (WGS) could be an overly excessive for "*targeted*" cases, thus being less effective in reaching a concrete diagnosis. By harnessing Whole Exome Sequencing (WES), several genes implicated in SCID may be analyzed simultaneously, thus providing a more thorough, cost-effective, and time-efficient method for obtaining a greater diagnostic yield.

3.2.1.5 Whole Genome Sequencing

Whole Genome Sequencing (WGS) is a high-throughput approach for sequencing a person's whole genome, including protein-coding and non-coding regions as well as regulatory and retroelements [65]. While the centromeric and telomeric areas were previously underserved, current advances have improved this aspect [66]. Among all NGS approaches, WGS is the most comprehensive genomic test because it allows simultaneous testing of several variant types across multiple genes without the use of a capture probe library. Due to this property, WES is an appealing method for identifying people with PID [67] (see Box 3.5). In contrast to gene panels and WES, WGS maintains consistent read depth, usually 20-X to 30-X lower than WES, with the option to increase at a substantial cost (e.g., to 60-X). WGS preserves the benefits of WES while adding non-coding genomic coverage and the capacity to detect copy number variations (CNVs) owing to consistent read depth [10].

To use WGS and WES effectively, understanding how to filter sequencing data is necessary. In "narrowing down" candidate genes for PID, it is crucial to prioritize variants based on their impact on protein product sequences [68]. This approach can be performed by using databases such as Exondel [69] and FishingCNV [70], and to filter out common variants from public databases. Algorithms such as pVAAST [71] and VarScan 2 [72] can help "narrowing down" candidate gene lists, especially for single-family analyses. Employing prediction models, which are trained with known PID genes, enhances prioritization based on function, pathway, expression, and phenotype connections. Tools such as Gene Damage Index (GDI) [73] and FLAGS [74] refine results by reducing noise associated with irrelevant mutations.

Box 3.5 Case Study 4: Whole Genome Sequencing (WGS)—Unusual, Acute and Frequent Mucosal Leishmaniasis Caused by Hyper-IgM Syndrome

A 19-year-old man presented with a 6-months period of throat irritation as well as *Leishmania tropica* infections. Initial treatment with liposomal amphotericin B (LAB) resolved symptoms; however, the recurring relapses required intravenous immunoglobulin (IVIG) replacement because of low IgG levels [75]. Due to low IgG and IgA levels, decreased switching memory B cells, and no major T cell deficit or other causes of hypogammaglobulinemia, the first diagnosis was "*Common Variable Immunodeficiency*" (CVID) [76]. Despite this initial diagnostic work-up, the clinically major manifestation of *L. tropica* did not match to CVID or to the B-cell depletion. A pathogenic variant [c.31C>T, p. (Arg11*)] of the *CD40L* gene was discovered by whole-genome sequencing and then confirmed by Sanger sequencing. So, we can observe that in complex and uncommon immunodeficiencies such as Hyper IgM Syndrome, WGS is favored over WES or gene panels for the identification of novel mutations [77, 78]. This statement is made because WGA enables an in-depth analysis, which in turn reconciles diagnostic ambiguities and provides solutions in clinical scenarios in which alternative techniques such as gene panels, Sanger sequencing, or Whole Exome Sequencing have not been successful in yielding a clinically meaningful diagnosis.

3.3 Structural Bioinformatics and Immunodeficiency-Associated Proteins: Algorithms for B- and T-Cell Receptors and Immunogenicity Prediction

Structural bioinformatics is a discipline that employs databases and computational tools to investigate the molecular folding, evolution, binding interactions, and structure–function connections of macromolecules such as proteins, RNA, and DNA [79]. Structural bioinformatics is commonly used for molecular docking, dynamics, visualization, structure prediction, mutation analysis, interactions at the atomic level, catalytic and binding site prediction, and database development [80].

Molecular docking investigates the interactions between proteins and ligands that can lead to more stable structures. This method is used to predict how a ligand binds to its target locations [81]. Molecular dynamics is a subfield in structural bioinformatics that employs molecular mechanics to imitate how atomic and subatomic interactions occur in macromolecules, as well as the consequences of these interactions [82]. Molecular visualization is a technique that allows researchers to evaluate and interpret macromolecule dynamic structures using visualization models such as cartoons, lines, surfaces, and stick models [83]. Last, protein structure prediction aims to determine how the amino acid sequence in a protein obtains a three-dimensional arrangement. These disciplines are essential in drug discovery and development, and enzyme engineering processes [84].

In the field of immunology, epitope prediction methods for B- and T-cell receptors are the most common application of structural bioinformatics. According to its definition, an antigen is a molecule that binds to an antibody and triggers an immune response. Via its antigen-binding site (also known as the paratope), an antibody binds to a specific antigen amino acid sequence, which is referred to as an epitope [85]. Conformational epitopes interact with the paratope based on their three-dimensional conformation, which is in turn, determined by the surface characteristics and shape of the antigen. Linear epitopes refer to the particular arrangement of amino acids in a peptide or protein that a T-cell receptor or antibody recognizes [86].

Immunoglobulins (Ig) function as surface B-cell receptors (BCRs), which trigger the production of antibodies during plasma cell development [79]. T-cell epitope immunogenicity involves antigen-presenting cells that express Major Histocompatibility Complex (MHC) molecules and further presentation of linear epitopes to T cells. Predicting peptide-MHC binding is crucial for anticipating T-cell epitopes, with MHC-peptide binding being the most selective determinant [87].

Epitope prediction methods for B- and T-cell receptors enrich our understanding of immunological responses [79], which is critical for vaccine development [88], antibody production [89], and immunodiagnostics [90], especially in immunocompromised patients [91]. Below, we provide a detailed overview of several techniques and methods for predicting T-cell and B-cell epitopes.

3.3.1 T-Cell Epitope Prediction

Structure-based approaches use molecular dynamic simulations to predict the MHC-peptide structure and assess interactions [92]. Data-driven techniques, on the other hand, employ sequence motifs (SM) that mimic the amino acid preferences of MHC molecules at amino acid residue positions that often appear at certain sites in MHC I and II binding peptides, known as "anchor residues" [93]. These sequences originate from epitope databases, such as the Immune Epitope Database (IEDB) [94], "EPIMHC" [95], and AntiJen [96]. Below, we will provide a brief description of such databases.

Firstly, IEDB [94] integrates various MHC Class I prediction tools, including Artificial Neural Networks (ANN) [97], ARB [98], Signal Matrix Model (SMM) [99], NetMHCcons [100], and PickPocket [101]. It also provides resources for predicting MHC II binding affinity through methods, such as SMM-align [102], together with epitope conservancy tools [103]. Processing prediction tools assess epitope candidacy according to proteasome cleavage, MHC binding, and transporters associated with antigen processing (TAP) [104]. Secondly, EPIMHC [95] predicts MHC binding peptides from user-supplied protein searches, generating personalized motif matrices for enhanced accuracy. Thirdly, AntiJen integrates immunological and vaccine-related data, offering comprehensive search techniques. Motif matrices (MM) and Quantitative Affinity Matrices (QAMs) evaluate peptide-MHC binding. AntiJen [96] is an immunological and vaccine-related database, which combines kinetic, thermodynamic, and functional information. AntiJen includes knowledge of MHC, TCR, TAP peptide interactions, antibody binding, and protein–protein interactions. In addition, AntiJen provides biophysical information for immunological molecules and complexes, by encompassing diffusion coefficients, cell surface copy count, and position-specific peptide libraries.

Researchers use motif matrices (MM) to assess the impact of peptide positions on MHC binding without determining affinity values [105]. Quantitative Affinity Matrices (QAMs) are employed for predicting binding affinity; however, the QAMs and MM often presume an autonomous influence of peptide side chains, notwithstanding indications of interactions among neighboring residues. Of note, quantitative structure–activity relationship additive models have been applied to address this problem. These models consider the cumulative influence of amino acid contributions at each position, as well as interactions with adjacent side chains [106].

Nonlinear peptide-MHC binding data is efficiently managed by machine learning (ML) algorithms, based on datasets comprising peptides with known affinity to MHC molecules. Recent advancements enable these algorithms to distinguish between MHC binding and non-binding peptides and to predict peptide-MHC affinity [107]. Examples include: ML-based discriminative models such as artificial neural networks (ANNs) [108], support vector machines (SVMs) [109], and Hidden Markov models (HMMs) [110]. Combining various approaches and offering consensus predictions enhances the performance of peptide-MHC predictions [107].

A major obstacle in using peptide-MHC binding models to predict T-cell epitopes is the large number of HLA allelic variations [111]. To address this issue, a team of researchers has created "pan-MHC-specific" techniques using input data comprising peptide-interacting MHC residues as well as peptide-binding affinity to train artificial neural networks (ANNs) [112]. These techniques predict peptide-binding affinities for unidentified HLA alleles. Similarly, web-based approaches such as MULTIPRED [113] and PEPVAC [114] predict promiscuous peptide binding to HLA subtypes.

3.3.2 B-Cell Epitope Prediction

3.3.2.1 Prediction of Linear B-Cell Epitopes

Additional amino acid propensity scales, which consider flexibility, accessibility, and β-turn, have been integrated to anticipate B-cell epitopes [93]. Examples of these tools include: PREDITOP [115], PEOPLE [116], and the Kolaskar and Tongaonkar method [117], the latter of which employs an immunogenicity scale based on physicochemical parameters and amino acid frequencies in confirmed epitopes.

BepiPred [118] employs antigen sequences and incorporates. Numerical models from the ESM-2 model to increase the predictive accuracy of B-cell epitopes. It does so by utilizing a residue annotation process for those epitopes that are previously defined in past studies and, in turn, by meticulously determining the predictor's architecture, training approach, and supplemental input factors.

ABCpred [119] employs recurrent neural networks that were trained using B-cell epitopes registered in the database "Bcipep." ABCpred is expected to exhibit enhanced performance in predicting B-cell epitopes of antigens, achieving a 65.93% accuracy in predicting B-cell epitopes. ABCpred and similar methods encounter limitations, such as utilizing small datasets and random peptides as non-B-cell epitopes.

The LBtope [120] web server, which was crafted with 12,063 epitopes and 20,589 non-epitopes, uses various ML models, including support vector machines and k-nearest neighbors, to distinguish between epitopes and non-epitopes. The models achieved an accuracy of up to 86%, by utilizing a variety of features such as binary profiles, dipeptide composition, and amino acid pair profiles.

SVMtrip [121] uses the most recent sequencing data from the IEDB database [89] to propose a novel method of antigenic epitope prediction. To increase prediction performance, this method uses a Support Vector Machine (SVM) that integrates tri-peptide propensity and similarity scores, or SVMTriP. SVMTriP exhibits noteworthy precision at 55.2%, sensitivity at 80.1%, and an area under the curve (AUC) at 0.702.

3.3.2.2 Prediction of Conformational B-Cell Epitopes

DiscoTope [122], which is a B-cell epitope prediction program, excels by considering factors such as solvent exposure, amino acid statistics, and spatial details. It maintains robust prediction accuracy across resolved and anticipated structures, thus eliminating the need for experimental validation. Being available as both a web server and software, DiscoTope-3.0 accommodates up to 50 structures per submission, interacting seamlessly with RCSB [123] and AlphaFoldDB [124] to achieve comprehensive predictions on all reported proteins.

Researchers have also employed ML to predict conformational B-cell epitopes. EPITOPIA [125] computes an immunogenicity score for each residue exposed to the solvent using the 3D structure of the epitope as input. Alternatively, EPITOPIA scores each amino acid in the sequence if one is supplied. Furthermore, by applying color-coding immunogenicity ratings to either the amino acid sequence or the three-dimensional structure of the protein, the tool's powerful visualization function allows users to visually evaluate the immunogenicity of the protein under study.

CBTOPE [126] is a technique that utilizes the antigen's primary sequence to discover conformational B-cell epitopes without requiring the antigen's three-dimensional structure. Unlike previous methods, CBTOPE employs support vector machines (SVM) trained with characteristics unique to conformational B-cell epitopes from sequences and physicochemical data. This method demonstrates promise in epitope identification solely from the antigen's main sequence, achieving a remarkable 86.6% accuracy in cross-validation testing.

ElliPro [127] is an online tool that stands out due to its distinctive approach, incorporating an algorithm for residue clustering, such as MODELLER software [128], Jmol viewer, and Thornton's method. Thornton's method analyzes α-carbon coordinates and protein surfaces to identify antigens. This data is later associated with antigenic peptide factors (such as protrusion index, mobility, solvent accessibility, and hydrophilicity for prediction), which have been previously determined by experimental approaches [129]. ElliPro's antibody epitope prediction effectiveness was assessed using a standard data collection of conformational epitopes. ElliPro demonstrated superiority over several structure-oriented methods with an AUC value of 0.73. Last, PEPITO exhibits advanced performance by integrating scores based on amino acid propensity with exposure values across different distances in a half-sphere. Evaluation with the DiscoTope data revealed PEPITO achieved an AUC of 0.75 [130].

3.4 Data Integration and Multi-Omics Approaches in Immunology: Diagnostics and Biomarkers for Treatment Stratification

The combination of multiple *-omics* approaches, including genomics, transcriptomics, proteomics, and metabolomics (which can be potentially expanded in the future to lipidomics and glycomics) has nowadays enabled scientists and clinicians to understand the immune system and its dynamics at multiple levels compared to the past. This multidisciplinary approach has resulted in advancements in biomarkers' discovery for primary immunodeficiencies, facilitating the development of more precision medicine-based therapies [131, 132].

3.4.1 Single-Cell RNA Sequencing

Bulk RNA sequencing analyzes RNA from a large cell population, providing an average gene expression profile for the entire group; this approach offers insights into the collective behavior of gene expression [133]. In contrast, single-cell RNA sequencing (scRNA-seq) is a genomic technique designed to sequence the RNA of individual cells [134]. Bulk RNA sequencing and scRNA-seq have rather different workflows. On the one hand, bulk sequencing involves processing myriad cells at once, beginning with total RNA extraction and moving on to cDNA synthesis and high-throughput sequencing of the combined library. On the other hand, single-cell isolation, individual RNA extraction from each cell, and subsequent cDNA synthesis and library preparation are the procedures involved in scRNA-seq. The final high-throughput sequencing is carried out separately for the library of each cell [135].

In the context of immunology, scRNA-seq has been proven pivotal in identifying unique cell subsets crucial for specific immune cell types [136], revealing transcription factors [137], and signaling pathways vital for immune cell development [138]. This technique significantly enhances our comprehension of B-cell [139] and T-cell receptor sequences [140], quantitative gene expression data [141], and clonal diversity [142].

3.4.1.1 Single-Cell RNA Sequencing Pipeline

Single-Cell Isolation

The scRNA-seq process begins with isolating single cells and extracting their nucleic acid content. Isolation methods range from laser microdissection to fluorescence-activated cell sorting [143]. Subsequent steps involve standard techniques such as cell lysis, mRNA isolation, poly(A) + selection, and the crucial phases of reverse transcription and cDNA synthesis [144]. Conventional PCR or in vitro transcription can amplify cDNAs [145, 146]. Recent techniques have focused on either the 5′ or 3′ regions of transcripts to reduce the sequencing costs of profiling multiple cells. Incorporating Unique Molecular Identifiers (UMIs) or tags in the reverse

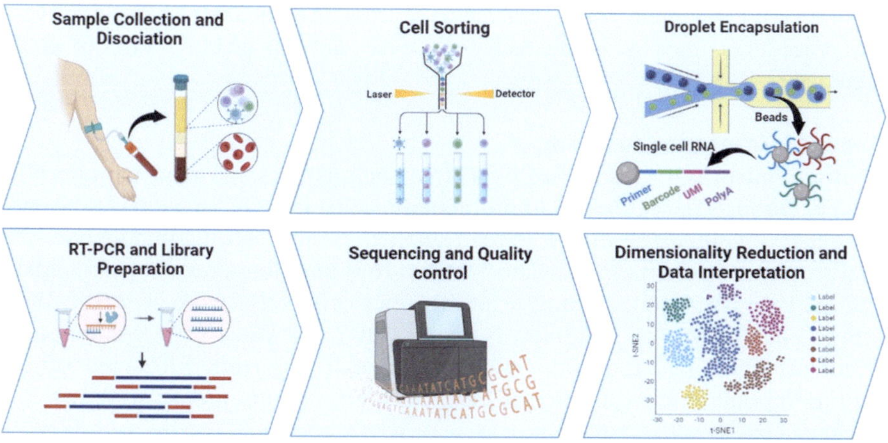

Fig. 3.2 Overview of single-cell RNA sequencing workflow. The process begins with the isolation of single cells from the target tissue or sample, by employing methods such as enzymatic digestion or fluorescence-activated cell sorting (FACS). Barcoding is then applied to uniquely label each cell, typically using molecular identifiers (UMIs) or cell-specific barcodes attached to RNA molecules. Following RNA extraction, reverse transcription, and library preparation, high-throughput sequencing generates comprehensive transcriptomic data for individual cells. Subsequent data preprocessing, quality control, and normalization steps ensure the reliability of the dataset. Unsupervised clustering algorithms are then employed to group cells based on gene expression profiles, revealing distinct cell populations and their heterogeneity. Cell types are identified through comparison with known markers or computational tools for cell type annotation. Differential gene expression analysis provides insights into the molecular mechanisms underlying immune responses, while functional analysis and data visualization techniques aid in understanding biological processes and relationships between cells. The results, which are visualized in reduced-dimensional spaces, offer a detailed transcriptional landscape of immune cells. This approach enables researchers to interpret individual cells' heterogeneity and functional states within the context of immunology. (Adapted from: Ona [148] and Kim et al. [149])

transcription stage simplifies molecular counting while improving accuracy by reducing PCR bias during the same process [147]. (See Fig. 3.2 for an overview of single-cell RNA sequencing workflow).

Reads Alignment

For scRNA-seq data, the mapping ratio, which serves as a crucial quality metric, is determined by read alignment efficiency. Tools like TopHat2 [150], STAR [151], and HISAT [152] are still relevant for scRNA-seq, with STAR known for its high algorithmic speed and HISAT for a balance between speed and accuracy. Spaced-seed indexing [153] and Burrows-Wheeler transform [154] are key read-mapping methods. Quantifying gene and transcript expression depends on the recorded transcript sequences, with whole-transcript approaches being applied in tools such as Smart-seq2 [155] and MATQ-seq [156]. Genome-guided assembly tools, such as Cufflinks [157], RSEM [158], and Stringtie [159], are frequently applied for transcript expression assessment, and they are recognized for superior reconstruction and quantification [160]. Unique molecular identifier (UMI)-based methods like

SAVER [161] are crucial for accurate gene expression estimation in 3′-end scRNA-seq procedures, thus reducing technical noise and enhancing transcript count accuracy.

Quality Control and Clustering

Quality control (QC) addresses concerns, such as bias and poor capture efficiency. Through the exclusion of problematic cells, FastQC checks for sequencing quality, while discarding low-read samples is an integral component of the quality control process [162]. The SinQC [163] and Scatter tools [164] calculate the expressed gene-to-transcript ratio per cell. ScRNA-seq-specific algorithms, such as Mutual Neighbor Network [165] and *k*-nearest neighbor batch effect test [166], manage common batch effects arising from differences attributed to the operator, experimental batches, spatial variation, and platform differences [167].

Using SCnorm [168], SAMstrt [169], and deconvolution-based algorithms [170], users can achieve normalization within or across samples. Imputation techniques, such as SAVER [161] and MAGIC [171], address missing data, incorporating spike-ins and UMIs. Statistical models, such as the Negative Binomial [172], address noise in single-cell differential expression analysis. Dimensionality reduction aims to simplify data visualization for the high-dimensional data obtained by scRNA-seq. Of note, *t*-distributed stochastic neighbor embedding (*t*-SNE) [173], Principal Component Analysis (PCA) [174], and Uniform Manifold Approximation and Projection (UMAP) [175] are those most frequent applied. Cell subpopulations are identified using techniques including graph-based clustering [176], density-based clustering [177], hierarchical clustering [178], and *k*-means [179]. These approaches apply clustering algorithms such as single-cell consensus clustering (SC3) [180] and Seurat [181]. The number of uninformative genes is decreased simultaneously by applying feature selection [182].

Differential Gene Expression

In single-cell RNA sequencing, identifying differently expressed genes (DEGs) across multiple cell subpopulations is essential. The issues of excessive noise, significant sample sizes, and technical heterogeneity in scRNA-seq data have led to the creation of sophisticated approaches, such as MAST [183], SCDE [184], DEsingle [185], Census [186], and BCseq [162]. All of the latter employ Bayesian techniques and linear model fitting, which are specifically designed for the particularities of scRNA-seq data compared to those of bulk RNA sequencing.

Regulatory Networks Inference

Understanding gene regulation networks (GRNs) is vital for linking genotypes to phenotypes. scRNA-seq enhances GRN analysis by capturing thousands of cells, and by overcoming challenges of gene–gene interactions and intracellular heterogeneity. Computational algorithms, including information theory techniques, facilitate assumption-free GRN inference. Incorporating stochastic aspects specific to single-cell data is crucial [187, 188].

Despite obstacles such as technical noise, scRNA-seq allows for discovering regulatory links and statistical heterogeneity, especially in T-cell biology. The variability of T cells is captured by scRNA-seq, whose data can provide valuable information on the unique roles and regulatory schemes of T cells [189]. scRNA-seq also reveals the molecular processes dictating T-cell fate decisions by identifying important regulators and signaling channels [190]. In addition, refining network directionality requires perturbation experiments or time-based information for causality inference [191].

3.4.2 Proteomics and Metabolomics

Proteomics and metabolomics significantly enhance our comprehension of translational immunology. Proteomics studies the entire protein complement in specific conditions, revealing immune subtleties through large-scale protein expression analysis [192], while metabolomics explore the entire set of metabolites in an organism, thus offering insights into immune cell metabolic landscapes and their impact on function [193].

3.4.2.1 MS-Omics Pipeline

Mass spectrometry (MS) is the gold standard in proteomic and metabolomic analyses. The preparation of samples for mass spectrum analysis aims to efficiently extract target analytes and to eliminate contaminants using filters to distinguish proteins from other substances according to their molecular weight, hydrophilicity, charge, or specific affinity [194]. Chromatography introduces analytes to the mass detector based on chemical-physical characteristics. The mobile phase transports analytes into the mass spectrometer, while the stationary phase separates them. Electrospray ionization (ESI) is widely used in molecular biology for its versatility in ionizing several analytes, and it enables the identification of analytes by the mass spectrometer [195]. Other ionization methods encompass electron ionization [196], matrix-assisted laser desorption ionization [197], and atmospheric-pressure chemical ionization [198].

By recording the ratio between mass and charge of charged particles, the mass spectrometer captures essential data for analysis, and it provides snapshots of precursor ions at a specific retention time (RT) in a single scan [199]. Table 3.3 presents

Table 3.3 Methods for chromatography-mass spectrometry integration

Method	Description
Liquid chromatography coupled with mass spectrometry (LC-MS)	Separation based on hydrophilicity, charge, size, or affinities. Identifies and quantifies compounds in complex mixtures [200]
Gas chromatography coupled with mass spectrometry (GC-MS)	Analyses volatile and semi-volatile compounds by separation based on polarity [201]
Capillary electrophoresis coupled with mass spectrometry (CE-MS)	Analyses biomolecules, peptides, and proteins based on separation by size, charge, and flow resistance [202]

the methods, and a description of the associated principles, separation mechanisms, and applications for combining chromatography and mass spectrometry.

Raw data refers to vendor-exclusive formats, converted to open formats using converters. Users commonly utilize NetCDF (Network Common Data Format) [203], MzXML [204], and the XML standard [205], Annotated Putative Peptide Markup Language (APML) [206], in order to create individual files containing both the original data and additional modifications. Algorithms use raw data for feature detection and noise reduction, and they require conversion from proprietary formats to accessible types. Processes such as noise reduction, peak-picking, feature identification, deisotoping, and deconvolution precede analyte identification; however, they present unresolved challenges [207]. Analyte identification involves comparing experimental features with theoretical patterns in databases [208, 209].

3.4.3 Metagenomics: The Microbiome in Primary Immunodeficiencies

Metagenomics employs next-generation sequencing techniques to study microbial nucleic acids extracted from clinical samples. Rather than relying on clonal cultures for classical microbial genome sequencing, early-stage metagenomic next-generation sequencing aimed to provide a diversity profile in a natural sample by commonly using the highly abundant 16S rRNA gene [210].

Nowadays, metagenomic shotgun next-generation sequencing (mNGS) is crucial for enhancing patient care and diagnostics in PIDs since patients with PIDs may suffer from infections caused by microbes that are not atypical or not detected by standard methods. Indeed, the objective of the above method is to identify atypical pathogens, a process that is clinically vital for PIDs with challenging microorganisms [211]. Metagenomics excels at revealing polymicrobial infections or those due to unculturable microbes or viruses and informing treatment decisions by identifying genetic markers of drug resistance. Also, its culture-free nature appears to be advantageous for patients receiving antibiotics. Additionally, metagenomics aids in the continuous monitoring of patients with PID, supporting ongoing research and promising improved outcomes and diagnostic accuracy [212].

Using primers derived from conserved genes such as ribosomal RNA (rRNA), the universal PCR technique facilitates the precise identification of bacteria, fungi, parasites, and other pathogens, even at the genus or species level [213]. In contrast, shotgun sequencing can perform both host and microbial nucleic acids without the need for specialized primers and probes. With the difficulty of distinguishing pathogen reads from the great majority of human host reads, clinical metagenomics concentrates on the identification of a wide variety of pathogens versus human host transcriptome profiling [214]. The incorporation of magnetic beads in the probe capture enrichment steps improves the efficiency in targeted mNGS of microbes and gene libraries. These methods provide flexible choices for pathogen detection, microbiome analysis, and host transcriptomic profiles, and they are compatible with

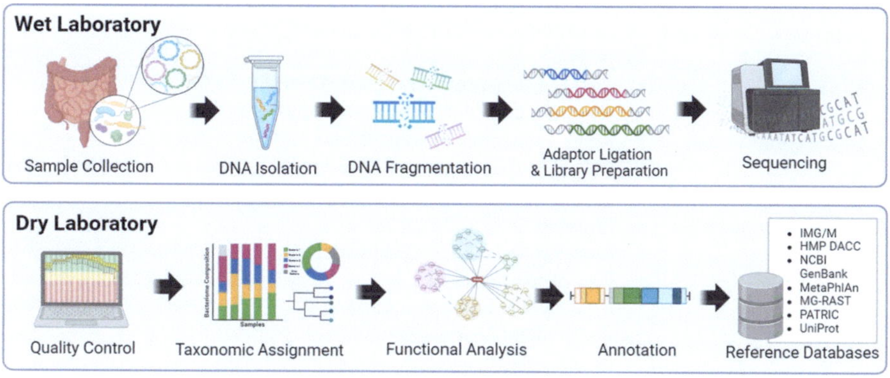

Fig. 3.3 Overview of metagenomics NGS wet and dry laboratory workflow. The mNGS workflow starts with collecting clinical specimens, such as tissues or body fluids, and progresses to DNA extraction, which isolates genetic material. Further, the library preparation generates small DNA fragments, which are then ligated to adapters, allowing for high-throughput NGS sequencing. Data processing and quality control ensure that raw sequencing data is reliable and clinically relevant. In the following steps, bioinformatics techniques are used for taxonomic assignment, revealing the exact microbial species found in patient samples. This involves comparing the data to reference databases. Furthermore, functional annotation enables the prediction of microbial functional functions by comparing sequences to databases containing clinically significant genes. Statistical techniques are then used for community analysis, allowing to investigate microbial composition and abundance in patient-specific microbiomes. The next phase requires biological interpretation of results in the clinical setting, which includes identifying significant microbial elements that may have an impact on patient health, therapy, or diagnosis (Adapted from: Castañeda-Mogollón et al. [216] and Dash and Das [217]). *Abbreviations*: *IMG/M* Integrated Microbial Genomes with Microbiome Samples; *HMP DACC* Human Microbiome Project Data Analysis and Coordination Center; *NCBI GenBank, MetaPhlAn* Metagenomic Phylogenetic Analysis; *MG-RAST* Metagenomics Rapid Annotation using Subsystem Technology; *PATRIC* Pathosystems Resource Integration Center; and UniProt

both portable nanopore sequencers and conventional benchtop devices [215]. (See Fig. 3.3 for an overview of metagenomics NGS wet and dry laboratory workflow).

3.4.4 Identification of Biomarkers for Patient Stratification

A biomarker is an assessable feature which is used to predict biological processes, diseases, or treatment outcomes. During the discovery phase, researchers examine candidate biomarkers that are associated with a disease or treatment using accessible samples, which most often consist of bodily fluids. Numerous candidates emerge during that process, each requiring validation before proceeding to clinical investigations. Validation includes assay development to ensure sensitivity and selectivity for monitoring specific biomarkers [218]. Key biomarkers related to cellular behavior, cytokine responses, systemic immune activities, and chronic immunological activation are listed in Table 3.4.

Table 3.4 Biomarkers for primary immunodeficiency

Biomarker type	Biomarkers
mRNA	• Elevated IFN-responsive genes [219] • Decrease in B- and T-cell transcripts [219]
Cellular components	• Reduced memory B cells [220] • Increased CD21-negative B cells [221–223] • Decreased naive and regulatory T cells [224–226]
Cytokine biomarkers	• Elevated TNF-α [227, 228] • Elevated IFN-γ [229–231] • IL-2 insufficiency [232] • B-cell activating factor [233] • B-cell maturation antigen [234] • Serum IgM levels [234, 235]
Other biomarkers	• High-density lipoprotein (HDL) [236] • Human lipopolysaccharide (LPS)-binding protein (LBP) [237] • sCD25 [238]

3.5 Bioinformatics for Drug Discovery in Primary Immunodeficiencies

The use of AI in bioinformatics significantly simplifies drug research, lowers costs, shortens time to market, and guarantees affordable access to effective medications [239]. Genetic mutations in hematopoietic cells frequently cause PIDs. Hematopoietic Stem Cell Transplantation (HSCT) replaces faulty hematopoietic stem cells with healthy donor cells [240]. Bioinformatics tools use algorithms to examine human leukocyte antigen (HLA) markers to analyze the genetic profiles of potential donors and recipients [241, 242]. Novel tools predict the chance of a donor matching a certain patient using HLA haplotype frequencies based on a variety of matching criteria. Table 3.5 lists several computational tools with comprehensive descriptions of their characteristics and functionalities which are intended to optimize the donor search procedure in HLA-matching.

3.5.1 Gene Therapy Approaches

Gene therapies most frequently utilize viral vectors to deliver therapeutic genes into a patient's cells, aiming to correct or replace altered genes to ultimately address the underlying genetic causes of diseases. The procedure involves treating blood stem cells from patients with a specific mutation, most frequently by using a retroviral vector, in order to integrate a non-pathogenic gene into the host cell genome. The reintroduction of the repaired gene is particularly valuable when an HLA-related donor is unavailable, thus reducing the risks associated with allogenic HSCT conditioning regimens and preventing graft-versus-host events [248].

Machine learning tied to bioinformatics aims to revolutionize the development of gene therapy. In particular, customized medicines can be made possible by anticipating and optimizing responses to gene-based therapeutics

Table 3.5 HLA-matching tools for donor search optimization

Tool	Description
DKMS Hap-E Search [243]	• Efficiently searches seven million donors • Provides precise 10/10 and 9/10 match probabilities • Data preparation: 1–2 days initially, <9 min/day for updates • Scalable for large donor databases
ZKRD OptiMatch® [244]	• Search engine based on serology-to-DNA mapping • Calculates allele-level matching based on German population frequencies • Web-based front end for extensive configuration • Robust security architecture
French Donor Registry EasyMatch® [245]	• Leverages haplotype frequencies for donor searches • Reduces costs and delays • Facilitates tracking of mismatches and estimates potential donors • Enables population selection based on patients' ethnic origin • Reliable predictions for high or low probabilities
HapLogic Algorithm [246]	• Predictive HLA-matching for unrelated donors and umbilical cord blood • Considers serologic and DNA typing equivalency • Locus-specific predictions with high accuracy • Ongoing research for enhancements • AUC values reflect high accuracy
HaploStats R Package [247]	• Used to investigate genetic variants and links to phenotypic characteristics or illnesses in haplotype-based association studies • Includes estimation of haplotype frequencies, association testing for genetic variations, and visualization tools for analyzing results

[249–251]. Driven by bioinformatics and artificial intelligence, predictive pre-clinical analysis can predict outcomes with higher accuracy compared to standard approaches, thus speeding up drug development options. Such approaches also advance the individualization of therapy, and transform the search for safer, more potent medications. Regarding PIDs, predictive pre-clinical analysis locates genetic variants, which is an essential approach for developing targeted gene treatments and improving therapy for primary immunodeficiency (PID). By assessing immune responses and directing specialized cell-based therapy, this technique can assist patients with PID in receiving personalized cellular therapies. In addition, AI-based models have been used to predict treatment outcomes in patients with primary immunodeficiencies [252]. In particular, Wang et al. used machine learning algorithms to calculate the risk factors associated with early mortality after umbilical cord blood transplantation in children with inborn errors of immunity. The model showed an area under the curve of 0.738 and successfully identified pre-transplant serum albumin levels, pre-transplant absolute CD4-positive lymphocyte count, high levels of c-reactive protein, and previous sepsis as predictors of early mortality. Such approaches facilitate medical decision-making, optimize therapeutic strategies, and allow patients and their relatives to make informed decisions based on their risk levels for patients with PID [253].

3.5.2 Other Applications: Drug Repurposing and Protein Druggability

Repurposing drugs that have already been assessed in humans accelerates the transition to clinical usage, and it represents a financially sustainable strategy [254] (see Box 3.6). Bioinformatics approaches play a key role in this process by analyzing biological information and predicting therapeutic linkages using AI algorithms, such as Logistic Regression [255], and tools such as the DeepPurpose Toolkit [256]. Researchers often use causal frameworks to construct networks that illustrate the relationships between medications, illnesses, proteins, and genes. Novel algorithms such as Long Short-Term Memory Networks enable the use of real-world data analysis to assess confounders and reduce biases [257].

Protein druggability relies on a protein's ability to bind small drug-like compounds, which is a crucial factor in drug development. Enzymes with similar ligand-binding patterns assist in understanding drug function and potential inhibitors. In structure-based evaluations, 3D protein structures and computational approaches have been employed to discover binding pockets, with automated systems like DoGSiteScorer [258] predicting druggability. Also, network-based druggability in machine learning utilizes molecular interaction networks [259].

Box 3.6 Case Studies in Bioinformatics for Drug Discovery

Case 1: Revolutionizing RAG1-SCID Treatment Through Gene Therapy.

In a pioneering study addressing challenges in RAG1-SCID treatment, scientists developed a gene therapy strategy, in which they optimized the efficient delivery of the *RAG1* gene via lentiviral vectors based on bioinformatic calculations. Successful in vitro tests demonstrated precise cell transduction under defined conditions. In NSTM (normal homologous serum) mice, i.e., the most highly immunodeficient mice, transplantation techniques combined with busulfan conditioning resulted in effective immune reconstitution. A tool-based monitoring and analysis strategy for immune repertoire analysis, which assessed lentiviral insertion sites and evaluated overall safety and efficacy, showed notable benefits. Assessing the safety of vectors involved using an in vitro immortalization test, with additional support from bioinformatics tools. The outcomes demonstrated gene therapy's potential for RAG1 Severe Combined Immunodeficiency (SCID), and they highlighted how important is the use of bioinformatic tools to help with decision-making and navigating the intricacies involved in developing novel treatments [260].

Case 2: Theophylline as a Novel Drug for Activated Phosphatidylinositol 3-Kinase-Delta Syndrome.

By having analyzed multiple phenotypic (also known as "*phenome*") data, pathways, networks, and genomic and epigenetic associations, scientists investigated redesigned uses for already-approved drugs (a process also known as "*drug repurposing*"). In particular, computational studies have led to drug repurposing of theophylline as a medication for Activated Phosphatidylinositol 3 Kinase Delta Syndrome (APDS), which is an immunological condition that is associated with increased lymphoproliferation and susceptibility to infections. In this context, an 11-year-old female patient with APDS due to PIK3R1 mutation showed improvement after receiving theophylline medication. As theophylline efficiently inhibits phosphatidylinositol three kinase delta (PI3Kδ), this repurposed drug has shown its promise by reducing the rate of lymph node pathologies and infection rates. Therefore, the effective combination of insights and bioinformatics-driven drug repurposing highlights the benefits of precision medicine and collaborative computational research in managing immunodeficiency diseases [261].

Case 3: CTLA4-IgG Fusion Proteins Complexity Deciphered Using Bioinformatics.

Cytotoxic T-lymphocyte associated protein 4 (CTLA-4) is an immune checkpoint protein that inhibits active T-cells [262]. Lipopolysaccharide Responsive Beige-Like Anchor Protein (LRBA) is a chaperone for CTLA4, facilitating its endosomal-mediated recycling. Deficiencies of LRBA produce CTLA-4 degradation, which further leads to immunodeficiencies [263–265]. Researchers actively investigated the three-dimensional structure of CTLA-4 in a study of LRBA deficiency and CTLA-4 haploinsufficiency. This study involved employing structural bioinformatics approaches, such as homology modeling and molecular dynamics simulations, with a particular focus on the ligand-binding area affected by the mutation. Visualization tools such as PyMOL and Visual Molecular Dynamics (VMD) revealed changes in amino acid spatial arrangement, predicting potential effects on CTLA-4's interaction with CD80 and CD86 ligands. Tools such as PolyPhen, SIFT, and Protein Variation Effect Analyzer (PROVEAN) identified and prioritized potential contributions of the mutations to the autoimmune phenotype. Also, comparative genomics confirmed the evolutionary conservation of the mutant residue (Pro138) in CTLA-4 across species, thus highlighting its significance in CTLA-4 function and enhancing our understanding of autoimmune disorders. CTLA4-IgG therapeutic fusion proteins, such as abatacept and belatacept, caused a restoration in checkpoint levels and improvement of the symptoms in CTLA-4 and LRBA deficient individuals [266]. These fusion proteins offer a promising avenue for targeted treatment by restoring regulatory T-cell functions and addressing lymphoproliferative and inflammatory symptoms [267].

3.6 Future Directions in Computational Immunology: Artificial Intelligence and Machine Learning in Immunodeficiency Diagnosis

PID is difficult to diagnose due to its complicated genetic makeup and wide range of symptoms, which hinder standardizing diagnostic pathways [268]. Because of AI progress, computers can now mimic human brain activities, such as understanding, reasoning, generalization, and experience-based learning [269]. There are several ways to approach AI challenges, including supervised and unsupervised learning. Supervised learning utilizes labeled data for assessing algorithmic performance after training and validation; indeed, most techniques include some form of supervised learning. Testing involves evaluating algorithmic performance, variation, and bias on a hidden dataset [270].

ML is the process by which systems learn and integrate information by making a multitude of observations. ML chiefly works by acquiring new insights and evolving through learning rather than being specifically programmed with new knowledge [271]. Table 3.6 describes various machine learning algorithms, and it highlights their applications and significance in addressing diverse challenges, such as disease diagnosis, classification tasks, and regression analysis.

3.6.1 Applications of Artificial Intelligence in Primary Immunodeficiency Patient Care

By harnessing AI in patient care, the SPIRIT® Analyzer efficiently manages risk factors for primary immunodeficiency by employing machine learning algorithms to classify patients based on 60 million records. This groundbreaking tool, which

Table 3.6 Machine learning algorithms for classification and regression

Algorithm	Description
Decision Tree (DT) [272]	A predictive model that employs a tree-like structure to map input data to target values for regression and classification tasks. Widely used DT algorithms include C4.5 and EC4.5
Support Vector Machine (SVM) [273]	Machine learning approach for addressing classification and regression challenges. Its applications span from disease diagnosis, recognizing facial features and speech, to predicting protein folds and discovering homologies
K-Nearest Neighbor (KNN) [274]	Nonparametric classification technique for both classification and regression analysis. Utilizes Euclidean distance techniques for determining the distance between data samples
Naïve Bayes (NB) [275]	Bayesian-based probabilistic classifier. Predicts membership probability for each class centered on a previously established record or data point. Used to project likelihood instead of predictions
Logistic Regression (LR) [255]	Used to solve classification problems that employ the sigmoid function inside a probability frame, using estimated values between 0 and 1

has demonstrated flexibility and dependability in pilot testing across health plans, offers a forward-thinking approach to risk assessment and preemptive healthcare measures [276]. Rider et al. have employed SPIRIT® as an efficient AI solution for PI risk assessment to identify high-risk individuals. This flexible technique not only systematically measures individual-level PI risk but also improves healthcare value and facilitates early PI diagnosis, with 0.2% of participants receiving the diagnosis of PID [277].

Computable phenotypes are derived based on data derived from electronic health records (EHR), and they are essential for diagnosing clinical diseases and risk-stratifying PID diseases. An artificial intelligence (AI) prediction model implemented in EHRs effectively identified PID patients in the study by Mayampurath et al. The entire logistic regression (LR) model, which attempted to integrate comorbidities, test findings, and history data, revealed optimum discrimination. Importantly, the complete LR model displayed improved sensitivity and specificity compared to the partial LR model. The above emphasizes how important the inclusion of a variety of clinical symptoms is to accurately diagnose primary immunodeficiency disorders (PIDD) [278].

Shifting to probabilistic models, a recently developed Bayesian network (BN) appears to play a pivotal role in assessing the probability of PID. This BN algorithm integrates EHR claims data, ensuring automatic and efficient results in diagnostic evaluations [279]. Likewise, the inclusion of immunologic disease terminology in the "Human Phenotype Ontology" (HPO) [52] enables the linking of patients' features with genetic data. Combining laboratory data, genomic information, unstructured EHR data processed with NLP, HPO keywords, and networks in immunobiology, clinical, and laboratory domains leads collectively to creating digital phenotypes [280].

3.7 Current Challenges and Future Perspectives in Computational Immunology for Primary Immunodeficiencies

Despite its undeniable value and exponential potential, AI cannot substitute skilled physicians (especially during their contact and human "touch" with patients), while at the same time, skepticism arises from perceived algorithmic opaqueness as well as the need for robust clinical validation. Previous incidents, such as certain commercial algorithms' inaccurate cancer advice, have contributed to relevant concerns. In addition, implicit bias poses significant challenges, requiring diverse training data to mitigate disparities, while current healthcare inequalities impact the effectiveness of Clinical Decision Support (CDS) systems. Addressing bias and representation gaps is critical for AI to attain its full potential, including in clinical allergy and immunology [281].

PIDs confront integration issues due to procedure variances and patient variability. Genetic diversity, which contributes to "missing heritability," impedes prediction algorithms across populations. The intricacy of "genetic epistasis," a gene interaction where a gene expression is influenced by other genes [282] and other interactions between common and uncommon variants confound computational immunology models. Omitting uncommon variants causes research and potentially clinical gaps, hindering a thorough understanding of immunological dynamics. Genetic heterogeneity presents obstacles into "multi-omics" data integration, thus necessitating complicated analytical frameworks. Despite its potential, computational immunology struggles to translate research into applicable therapies, requiring collaborative efforts and innovative solutions for algorithm development, data integration, and genetic foundations to realize its full potential in explaining immune-related diseases [283].

In addition, predicting protein structures in computational biology has been challenging for more than 50 years. This difficulty is mainly due to the absence of distinguishing qualities or attributes linked with certain functions that, in turn, create a barrier to developing an algorithm. Anticipating detailed protein structures is critical for proper immune response modeling; as a result, the field has suboptimal precision in simulating immune-related processes that are impacted by mutations caused by environmental variables. Overcoming this barrier is critical for progressing computationally inspired medical immunology and for improving predictions of immune system behavior [284]. Projects such as the AlphaFold Protein Structure Database can illuminate protein prediction approaches [285].

Last but not least, the application of ML to rare diseases, and in this case, PIDs, faces obstacles due to information scarcity, the complexity of rare diseases, and prolonged diagnostic processes. Ethical, technological, and methodological challenges arise, requiring ML techniques to adapt to the limited data available on rare diseases. Legal issues, especially General Data Protection Regulation (GDPR) compliance, impact patient privacy. Disease registries, standardized data collection, and acknowledgment of open data are crucial; however, consistency issues still persist. Small sample sizes and data intensity necessitate techniques such as data augmentation. Ensuring explainability and fairness is vital. Federated ML offers a secure approach, which requires a collaborative strategy that will aim to address ethical, technical, and healthcare challenges for the successful application of ML approaches to rare diseases, such as PIDs [286].

Acknowledgments AFAM would like to thank Ms. Anna Gkika for her continuous moral support throughout this study.

Contributions AFAM conceived and contributed to the original idea and study design with input from JdMPM. JdPMV performed the initial literature review and drafted the initial version of the manuscript with input from AFAM. AFAM revised the manuscript for critical intellectual content based on the content initially drafted by JdPMV. Both authors approved the final version of the manuscript.

Conflicts of Interest AFAM has served as an employee of BGI Genomics. No financial or other conflicts of interest that could have exercised an influence on this work appear to exist.

References

1. Chang C (2022) Allergic and immunologic diseases: a practical guide to the evaluation, diagnosis, and management of allergic and immunologic diseases. Academic, London
2. Giardino G, Gallo V, Prencipe R et al (2016) Unbalanced immune system: immunodeficiencies and autoimmunity. Front Pediatr 4:107. https://doi.org/10.3389/fped.2016.00107
3. Ghosh S (2020) Computational immunology. Applications. CRC Press, Boca Raton, FL
4. Yska HAF, Elsink K, Kuijpers TW et al (2019) Diagnostic yield of next generation sequencing in genetically undiagnosed patients with primary immunodeficiencies: a systematic review. J Clin Immunol 39:577–591. https://doi.org/10.1007/s10875-019-00656-x
5. Van Schouwenburg PA, Davenport EE, Kienzler A-K et al (2015) Application of whole genome and RNA sequencing to investigate the genomic landscape of common variable immunodeficiency disorders. Clin Immunol 160:301–314. https://doi.org/10.1016/j.clim.2015.05.020
6. Stray-Pedersen A, Sorte HS, Samarakoon P et al (2017) Primary immunodeficiency diseases: genomic approaches delineate heterogeneous Mendelian disorders. J Allergy Clin Immunol 139:232–245. https://doi.org/10.1016/j.jaci.2016.05.042
7. Sanger F, Nicklen S, Coulson AR (1977) DNA sequencing with chain-terminating inhibitors. Proc Natl Acad Sci USA 74:5463–5467. https://doi.org/10.1073/pnas.74.12.5463
8. De Cario R, Kura A, Suraci S et al (2020) Sanger validation of high-throughput sequencing in genetic diagnosis: still the best practice? Front Genet 11:592588. https://doi.org/10.3389/fgene.2020.592588
9. Chan K-W, Wong C-Y, Leung D et al (2022) Targeted gene Sanger sequencing should remain the first-tier genetic test for children suspected to have the five common X-linked inborn errors of immunity. Front Immunol 13:883446. https://doi.org/10.3389/fimmu.2022.883446
10. Chinn IK, Orange JS (2020) A 2020 update on the use of genetic testing for patients with primary immunodeficiency. Expert Rev Clin Immunol 16:897–909. https://doi.org/10.1080/1744666X.2020.1814145
11. Aldave Becerra JC, Cachay Rojas E (2017) A 3-year-old girl with recurrent infections and autoimmunity due to a STAT1 gain-of-function mutation: the expanding clinical presentation of primary immunodeficiencies. Front Pediatr 5:55. https://doi.org/10.3389/fped.2017.00055
12. Eren Akarcan S, Ulusoy Severcan E, Edeer Karaca N et al (2017) Gain-of-function mutations in STAT1: a recently defined cause for chronic mucocutaneous candidiasis disease mimicking combined immunodeficiencies. Case Rep Immunol 2017:1–6. https://doi.org/10.1155/2017/2846928
13. Larson NB, Oberg AL, Adjei AA, Wang L (2023) A clinician's guide to bioinformatics for next-generation sequencing. J Thorac Oncol 18:143–157. https://doi.org/10.1016/j.jtho.2022.11.006
14. Next Generation Sequencing Workflow (2023). https://app.biorender.com/biorender-templates/figures/all/t-62ccc36459dc10d0850c42df-next-generation-sequencing-workflow
15. Lalrinmawii C, Muppalaneni NB (2023) An overview of the workflow of next-generation sequencing data analysis. In: 2023 4th international conference on electronics and sustainable communication systems (ICESC). IEEE, Coimbatore, India, pp 1655–1659
16. Clark DP, Pazdernik NJ, McGehee MR (2019) Molecular biology, 3rd edn. Academic Press, London, UK
17. Hu T, Chitnis N, Monos D, Dinh A (2021) Next-generation sequencing technologies: an overview. Hum Immunol 82:801–811. https://doi.org/10.1016/j.humimm.2021.02.012
18. Ardui S, Ameur A, Vermeesch JR, Hestand MS (2018) Single molecule real-time (SMRT) sequencing comes of age: applications and utilities for medical diagnostics. Nucleic Acids Res 46:2159–2168. https://doi.org/10.1093/nar/gky066
19. Wang Y, Zhao Y, Bollas A et al (2021) Nanopore sequencing technology, bioinformatics and applications. Nat Biotechnol 39:1348–1365. https://doi.org/10.1038/s41587-021-01108-x

20. Rothberg JM, Leamon JH (2008) The development and impact of 454 sequencing. Nat Biotechnol 26:1117–1124. https://doi.org/10.1038/nbt1485
21. Cock PJA, Fields CJ, Goto N et al (2010) The Sanger FASTQ file format for sequences with quality scores, and the Solexa/Illumina FASTQ variants. Nucleic Acids Res 38:1767–1771. https://doi.org/10.1093/nar/gkp1137
22. Li H (2013) Aligning sequence reads, clone sequences and assembly contigs with BWA-MEM. https://doi.org/10.48550/ARXIV.1303.3997
23. Langmead B, Salzberg SL (2012) Fast gapped-read alignment with Bowtie 2. Nat Methods 9:357–359. https://doi.org/10.1038/nmeth.1923
24. Lin H-N, Hsu W-L (2017) Kart: a divide-and-conquer algorithm for NGS read alignment. Bioinformatics 33:2281–2287. https://doi.org/10.1093/bioinformatics/btx189
25. Thankaswamy-Kosalai S, Sen P, Nookaew I (2017) Evaluation and assessment of read-mapping by multiple next-generation sequencing aligners based on genome-wide characteristics. Genomics 109:186–191. https://doi.org/10.1016/j.ygeno.2017.03.001
26. Li H (2018) Minimap2: pairwise alignment for nucleotide sequences. Bioinformatics 34:3094–3100. https://doi.org/10.1093/bioinformatics/bty191
27. Zhang H (2016) Overview of sequence data formats. In: Mathé E, Davis S (eds) Statistical genomics. Springer, New York, pp 3–17
28. Pedersen BS, Quinlan AR (2018) Mosdepth: quick coverage calculation for genomes and exomes. Bioinformatics 34:867–868. https://doi.org/10.1093/bioinformatics/btx699
29. Broad Institute Picard Tools. https://broadinstitute.github.io/picard/
30. Okonechnikov K, Conesa A, García-Alcalde F (2016) Qualimap 2: advanced multi-sample quality control for high-throughput sequencing data. Bioinformatics 32:292–294. https://doi.org/10.1093/bioinformatics/btv566
31. Ewels P, Magnusson M, Lundin S, Käller M (2016) MultiQC: summarize analysis results for multiple tools and samples in a single report. Bioinformatics 32:3047–3048. https://doi.org/10.1093/bioinformatics/btw354
32. Koboldt DC (2020) Best practices for variant calling in clinical sequencing. Genome Med 12:91. https://doi.org/10.1186/s13073-020-00791-w
33. Higasa K, Miyake N, Yoshimura J et al (2016) Human genetic variation database, a reference database of genetic variations in the Japanese population. J Hum Genet 61:547–553. https://doi.org/10.1038/jhg.2016.12
34. Tennessen JA, Bigham AW, O'Connor TD et al (2012) Evolution and functional impact of rare coding variation from deep sequencing of human exomes. Science 337:64–69. https://doi.org/10.1126/science.1219240
35. Sherry ST (2001) dbSNP: the NCBI database of genetic variation. Nucleic Acids Res 29:308–311. https://doi.org/10.1093/nar/29.1.308
36. McLaren W, Gil L, Hunt SE et al (2016) The Ensembl variant effect predictor. Genome Biol 17:122. https://doi.org/10.1186/s13059-016-0974-4
37. Wang K, Li M, Hakonarson H (2010) ANNOVAR: functional annotation of genetic variants from high-throughput sequencing data. Nucleic Acids Res 38:e164. https://doi.org/10.1093/nar/gkq603
38. DePristo MA, Banks E, Poplin R et al (2011) A framework for variation discovery and genotyping using next-generation DNA sequencing data. Nat Genet 43:491–498. https://doi.org/10.1038/ng.806
39. Beck TF, Mullikin JC, the NISC Comparative Sequencing Program, Biesecker LG (2016) Systematic evaluation of Sanger validation of next-generation sequencing variants. Clin Chem 62:647–654. https://doi.org/10.1373/clinchem.2015.249623
40. Belyeu JR, Chowdhury M, Brown J et al (2021) Samplot: a platform for structural variant visual validation and automated filtering. Genome Biol 22:161. https://doi.org/10.1186/s13059-021-02380-5
41. Liu Y, Yeung WSB, Chiu PCN, Cao D (2022) Computational approaches for predicting variant impact: an overview from resources, principles to applications. Front Genet 13:981005. https://doi.org/10.3389/fgene.2022.981005

42. Fang M, Su Z, Abolhassani H et al (2022) VIPPID: a gene-specific single nucleotide variant pathogenicity prediction tool for primary immunodeficiency diseases. Brief Bioinform 23:bbac176. https://doi.org/10.1093/bib/bbac176
43. Itan Y, Casanova J-L (2015) Novel primary immunodeficiency candidate genes predicted by the human gene connectome. Front Immunol 6:142. https://doi.org/10.3389/fimmu.2015.00142
44. Richards S, Aziz N, Bale S et al (2015) Standards and guidelines for the interpretation of sequence variants: a joint consensus recommendation of the American College of Medical Genetics and Genomics and the Association for Molecular Pathology. Genet Med 17:405–424. https://doi.org/10.1038/gim.2015.30
45. Karczewski KJ, Weisburd B, Thomas B et al (2017) The ExAC browser: displaying reference data information from over 60 000 exomes. Nucleic Acids Res 45:D840–D845. https://doi.org/10.1093/nar/gkw971
46. National Center for Biotechnology Information Variation Viewer. https://www.ncbi.nlm.nih.gov/variation/view/
47. The 1000 Genomes Project Consortium, Corresponding authors, Auton A et al (2015) A global reference for human genetic variation. Nature 526:68–74. https://doi.org/10.1038/nature15393
48. Chinn IK, Chan AY, Chen K et al (2020) Diagnostic interpretation of genetic studies in patients with primary immunodeficiency diseases: a working group report of the Primary Immunodeficiency Diseases Committee of the American Academy of Allergy, Asthma & Immunology. J Allergy Clin Immunol 145:46–69. https://doi.org/10.1016/j.jaci.2019.09.009
49. Landrum MJ, Chitipiralla S, Brown GR et al (2020) ClinVar: improvements to accessing data. Nucleic Acids Res 48:D835–D844. https://doi.org/10.1093/nar/gkz972
50. Lozano-Kühne J (2013) Disease databases. In: Dubitzky W, Wolkenhauer O, Cho K-H, Yokota H (eds) Encyclopedia of systems biology. Springer, New York, pp 575–577
51. Hamosh A (2004) Online Mendelian Inheritance in Man (OMIM), a knowledgebase of human genes and genetic disorders. Nucleic Acids Res 33:D514–D517. https://doi.org/10.1093/nar/gki033
52. Köhler S, Gargano M, Matentzoglu N et al (2021) The human phenotype ontology in 2021. Nucleic Acids Res 49:D1207–D1217. https://doi.org/10.1093/nar/gkaa1043
53. Cano-Gamez E, Trynka G (2020) From GWAS to function: using functional genomics to identify the mechanisms underlying complex diseases. Front Genet 11:424. https://doi.org/10.3389/fgene.2020.00424
54. The UniProt Consortium (2019) UniProt: a worldwide hub of protein knowledge. Nucleic Acids Res 47:D506–D515. https://doi.org/10.1093/nar/gky1049
55. Paysan-Lafosse T, Blum M, Chuguransky S et al (2023) InterPro in 2022. Nucleic Acids Res 51:D418–D427. https://doi.org/10.1093/nar/gkac993
56. Waterhouse A, Bertoni M, Bienert S et al (2018) SWISS-MODEL: homology modelling of protein structures and complexes. Nucleic Acids Res 46:W296–W303. https://doi.org/10.1093/nar/gky427
57. Cifaldi C, Brigida I, Barzaghi F et al (2019) Targeted NGS platforms for genetic screening and gene discovery in primary immunodeficiencies. Front Immunol 10:316. https://doi.org/10.3389/fimmu.2019.00316
58. Saudi Mendeliome Group (2015) Comprehensive gene panels provide advantages over clinical exome sequencing for Mendelian diseases. Genome Biol 16:134. https://doi.org/10.1186/s13059-015-0693-2
59. Rae W, Ward D, Mattocks C et al (2018) Clinical efficacy of a next-generation sequencing gene panel for primary immunodeficiency diagnostics. Clin Genet 93:647–655. https://doi.org/10.1111/cge.13163
60. Labrador-Horrillo M, Franco-Jarava C, Garcia-Prat M et al (2022) Case report: X-linked SASH3 deficiency presenting as a common variable immunodeficiency. Front Immunol 13:881206. https://doi.org/10.3389/fimmu.2022.881206

61. Vorsteveld EE, Hoischen A, Van Der Made CI (2021) Next-generation sequencing in the field of primary immunodeficiencies: current yield, challenges, and future perspectives. Clin Rev Allerg Immunol 61:212–225. https://doi.org/10.1007/s12016-021-08838-5
62. Platt CD, Zaman F, Bainter W et al (2021) Efficacy and economics of targeted panel versus whole-exome sequencing in 878 patients with suspected primary immunodeficiency. J Allergy Clin Immunol 147:723–726. https://doi.org/10.1016/j.jaci.2020.08.022
63. Simon AJ, Golan AC, Lev A et al (2020) Whole exome sequencing (WES) approach for diagnosing primary immunodeficiencies (PIDs) in a highly consanguineous community. Clin Immunol 214:108376. https://doi.org/10.1016/j.clim.2020.108376
64. Yan L, He Y, Zhang Y et al (2023) A novel 268 kb deletion combined with a splicing variant in IL7R causes of severe combined immunodeficiency in a Chinese family: a case report. BMC Med Genet 16:323. https://doi.org/10.1186/s12920-023-01765-8
65. Aspden JL, Wallace EWJ, Whiffin N (2023) Not all exons are protein coding: addressing a common misconception. Cell Genomics 3:100296. https://doi.org/10.1016/j.xgen.2023.100296
66. Nurk S, Koren S, Rhie A et al (2022) The complete sequence of a human genome. Science 376:44–53. https://doi.org/10.1126/science.abj6987
67. Lappalainen T, Scott AJ, Brandt M, Hall IM (2019) Genomic analysis in the age of human genome sequencing. Cell 177:70–84. https://doi.org/10.1016/j.cell.2019.02.032
68. Fang M, Abolhassani H, Lim CK et al (2016) Next generation sequencing data analysis in primary immunodeficiency disorders—future directions. J Clin Immunol 36:68–75. https://doi.org/10.1007/s10875-016-0260-y
69. Guo Y, Zhao S, Lehmann BD et al (2014) Detection of internal exon deletion with exon Del. BMC Bioinformatics 15:332. https://doi.org/10.1186/1471-2105-15-332
70. Shi Y, Majewski J (2013) FishingCNV: a graphical software package for detecting rare copy number variations in exome-sequencing data. Bioinformatics 29:1461–1462. https://doi.org/10.1093/bioinformatics/btt151
71. Hu H, Roach JC, Coon H et al (2014) A unified test of linkage analysis and rare-variant association for analysis of pedigree sequence data. Nat Biotechnol 32:663–669. https://doi.org/10.1038/nbt.2895
72. Koboldt DC, Larson DE, Wilson RK (2013) Using VarScan 2 for germline variant calling and somatic mutation detection. CP Bioinformatics 44:15.4.1. https://doi.org/10.1002/0471250953.bi1504s44
73. Itan Y, Shang L, Boisson B et al (2015) The human gene damage index as a gene-level approach to prioritizing exome variants. Proc Natl Acad Sci USA 112:13615–13620. https://doi.org/10.1073/pnas.1518646112
74. Shyr C, Tarailo-Graovac M, Gottlieb M et al (2014) FLAGS, frequently mutated genes in public exomes. BMC Med Genet 7:64. https://doi.org/10.1186/s12920-014-0064-y
75. Drabe CH, Marvig RL, Borgwardt L et al (2020) Case report: hyper IgM syndrome identified by whole genome sequencing in a young Syrian man presenting with atypical, severe and recurrent mucosal Leishmaniasis. Front Immunol 11:567856. https://doi.org/10.3389/fimmu.2020.567856
76. Seidel MG, Kindle G, Gathmann B et al (2019) The European Society for Immunodeficiencies (ESID) Registry working definitions for the clinical diagnosis of inborn errors of immunity. J Allergy Clin Immunol Pract 7:1763–1770. https://doi.org/10.1016/j.jaip.2019.02.004
77. Kiani-Alikhan S, Yong PFK, Gilmour KC et al (2012) Phenotypic heterogeneity in a family with a CD40 ligand intracellular domain mutation. J Clin Immunol 32:70–77. https://doi.org/10.1007/s10875-011-9607-6
78. Seyama K, Kobayashi R, Hasle H et al (1998) Parvovirus B19-induced anemia as the presenting manifestation of X-linked hyper-IgM syndrome. J Infect Dis 178:318–324. https://doi.org/10.1086/515633
79. Akcapinar GB, Sezerman OU (2017) Computational approaches for de novo design and redesign of metal-binding sites on proteins. Biosci Rep 37:BSR20160179. https://doi.org/10.1042/BSR20160179

80. Paiva VDA, Gomes IDS, Monteiro CR et al (2022) Protein structural bioinformatics: an overview. Comput Biol Med 147:105695. https://doi.org/10.1016/j.compbiomed.2022.105695
81. Morris GM, Lim-Wilby M (2008) Molecular docking. In: Kukol A (ed) Molecular modeling of proteins. Humana, Totowa, NJ, pp 365–382
82. Karplus M, McCammon JA (2002) Molecular dynamics simulations of biomolecules. Nat Struct Biol 9:646–652. https://doi.org/10.1038/nsb0902-646
83. Li H, Wei X (2024) A concise review of biomolecule visualization. CIMB 46:1318–1334. https://doi.org/10.3390/cimb46020084
84. Huang B, Kong L, Wang C et al (2023) Protein structure prediction: challenges, advances, and the shift of research paradigms. Genomics Proteomics Bioinformatics. https://doi.org/10.1016/j.gpb.2022.11.014
85. Murphy K, Weaver C (2016) Janeway's immunobiology, 9th edn. Garland Science/Taylor & Francis Group, LLC, New York
86. Bukhari SNH, Jain A, Haq E et al (2022) Machine learning techniques for the prediction of B-cell and T-cell epitopes as potential vaccine targets with a specific focus on SARS-CoV-2 pathogen: a review. Pathogens 11:146. https://doi.org/10.3390/pathogens11020146
87. Peters B, Nielsen M, Sette A (2020) T cell epitope predictions. Annu Rev Immunol 38:123–145. https://doi.org/10.1146/annurev-immunol-082119-124838
88. Soria-Guerra RE, Nieto-Gomez R, Govea-Alonso DO, Rosales-Mendoza S (2015) An overview of bioinformatics tools for epitope prediction: implications on vaccine development. J Biomed Inform 53:405–414. https://doi.org/10.1016/j.jbi.2014.11.003
89. Potocnakova L, Bhide M, Pulzova LB (2016) An introduction to B-cell epitope mapping and in silico epitope prediction. J Immunol Res 2016:1–11. https://doi.org/10.1155/2016/6760830
90. Goyal B, Kumar K, Gupta D et al (2014) Utility of B-cell epitopes based peptides of RD1 and RD2 antigens for immunodiagnosis of pulmonary tuberculosis. Diagn Microbiol Infect Dis 78:391–397. https://doi.org/10.1016/j.diagmicrobio.2013.12.018
91. Ahmed S, Rahman MN, Hasan M et al (2023) Immunogenic multi-epitope-based vaccine development to combat cyclosporiasis of immunocompromised patients applying computational biology method. Exp Parasitol 248:108497. https://doi.org/10.1016/j.exppara.2023.108497
92. Patronov A, Doytchinova I (2013) T-cell epitope vaccine design by immunoinformatics. Open Biol 3:120139. https://doi.org/10.1098/rsob.120139
93. Sanchez-Trincado JL, Gomez-Perosanz M, Reche PA (2017) Fundamentals and methods for T- and B-cell epitope prediction. J Immunol Res 2017:1–14. https://doi.org/10.1155/2017/2680160
94. Vita R, Mahajan S, Overton JA et al (2019) The Immune Epitope Database (IEDB): 2018 update. Nucleic Acids Res 47:D339–D343. https://doi.org/10.1093/nar/gky1006
95. Reche PA, Zhang H, Glutting J-P, Reinherz EL (2005) EPIMHC: a curated database of MHC-binding peptides for customized computational vaccinology. Bioinformatics 21:2140–2141. https://doi.org/10.1093/bioinformatics/bti269
96. Toseland CP, Clayton DJ, McSparron H et al (2005) AntiJen: a quantitative immunology database integrating functional, thermodynamic, kinetic, biophysical, and cellular data. Immunome Res 1:4. https://doi.org/10.1186/1745-7580-1-4
97. Nielsen M, Lundegaard C, Worning P et al (2003) Reliable prediction of T-cell epitopes using neural networks with novel sequence representations. Protein Sci 12:1007–1017. https://doi.org/10.1110/ps.0239403
98. Bui H-H, Sidney J, Peters B et al (2005) Automated generation and evaluation of specific MHC binding predictive tools: ARB matrix applications. Immunogenetics 57:304–314. https://doi.org/10.1007/s00251-005-0798-y
99. Peters B, Sette A (2005) Generating quantitative models describing the sequence specificity of biological processes with the stabilized matrix method. BMC Bioinformatics 6:132. https://doi.org/10.1186/1471-2105-6-132

100. Karosiene E, Lundegaard C, Lund O, Nielsen M (2012) NetMHCcons: a consensus method for the major histocompatibility complex class I predictions. Immunogenetics 64:177–186. https://doi.org/10.1007/s00251-011-0579-8
101. Zhang H, Lund O, Nielsen M (2009) The PickPocket method for predicting binding specificities for receptors based on receptor pocket similarities: application to MHC-peptide binding. Bioinformatics 25:1293–1299. https://doi.org/10.1093/bioinformatics/btp137
102. Nielsen M, Lundegaard C, Lund O (2007) Prediction of MHC class II binding affinity using SMM-align, a novel stabilization matrix alignment method. BMC Bioinformatics 8:238. https://doi.org/10.1186/1471-2105-8-238
103. Bui H-H, Sidney J, Li W et al (2007) Development of an epitope conservancy analysis tool to facilitate the design of epitope-based diagnostics and vaccines. BMC Bioinformatics 8:361. https://doi.org/10.1186/1471-2105-8-361
104. Tenzer S, Peters B, Bulik S et al (2005) Modeling the MHC class I pathway by combining predictions of proteasomal cleavage,TAP transport and MHC class I binding. Cell Mol Life Sci 62:1025–1037. https://doi.org/10.1007/s00018-005-4528-2
105. Desai DV, Kulkarni-Kale U (2014) T-cell epitope prediction methods: an overview. In: De RK, Tomar N (eds) Immunoinformatics. Springer, New York, pp 333–364
106. Tomar N, De RK (2010) Immunoinformatics: an integrated scenario. Immunology 131:153–168. https://doi.org/10.1111/j.1365-2567.2010.03330.x
107. Mukhopadhyay M (2023) Machine learning for MHC II specificities. Nat Methods 20:632–632. https://doi.org/10.1038/s41592-023-01891-2
108. Agatonovic-Kustrin S, Beresford R (2000) Basic concepts of artificial neural network (ANN) modeling and its application in pharmaceutical research. J Pharm Biomed Anal 22:717–727. https://doi.org/10.1016/S0731-7085(99)00272-1
109. Burges CJC (1998) A tutorial on support vector machines for pattern recognition. Data Min Knowl Disc 2:121–167. https://doi.org/10.1023/A:1009715923555
110. Eddy SR (1996) Hidden Markov models. Curr Opin Struct Biol 6:361–365. https://doi.org/10.1016/S0959-440X(96)80056-X
111. Nielsen M, Andreatta M, Peters B, Buus S (2020) Immunoinformatics: predicting peptide–MHC binding. Annu Rev Biomed Data Sci 3:191–215. https://doi.org/10.1146/annurev-biodatasci-021920-100259
112. Leman JK, Mueller R, Karakas M et al (2013) Simultaneous prediction of protein secondary structure and transmembrane spans. Proteins 81:1127–1140. https://doi.org/10.1002/prot.24258
113. Zhang GL, Khan AM, Srinivasan KN et al (2005) MULTIPRED: a computational system for prediction of promiscuous HLA binding peptides. Nucleic Acids Res 33:W172–W179. https://doi.org/10.1093/nar/gki452
114. Reche PA, Reinherz EL (2005) PEPVAC: a web server for multi-epitope vaccine development based on the prediction of supertypic MHC ligands. Nucleic Acids Res 33:W138–W142. https://doi.org/10.1093/nar/gki357
115. Pellequer JL, Westhof E (1993) PREDITOP: a program for antigenicity prediction. J Mol Graph 11:204–210. https://doi.org/10.1016/0263-7855(93)80074-2
116. Alix AJP (1999) Predictive estimation of protein linear epitopes by using the program PEOPLE. Vaccine 18:311–314. https://doi.org/10.1016/S0264-410X(99)00329-1
117. Kolaskar AS, Tongaonkar PC (1990) A semi-empirical method for prediction of antigenic determinants on protein antigens. FEBS Lett 276:172–174. https://doi.org/10.1016/0014-5793(90)80535-Q
118. Clifford JN, Høie MH, Deleuran S et al (2022) BepiPred-3.0: improved B-cell epitope prediction using protein language models. Protein Sci 31:e4497. https://doi.org/10.1002/pro.4497
119. Malik AA, Ojha SC, Schaduangrat N, Nantasenamat C (2022) ABCpred: a webserver for the discovery of acetyl- and butyryl-cholinesterase inhibitors. Mol Divers 26:467–487. https://doi.org/10.1007/s11030-021-10292-6

120. Singh H, Ansari HR, Raghava GPS (2013) Improved method for linear B-cell epitope prediction using antigen's primary sequence. PLoS One 8:e62216. https://doi.org/10.1371/journal.pone.0062216
121. Yao B, Zhang L, Liang S, Zhang C (2012) SVMTriP: a method to predict antigenic epitopes using support vector machine to integrate tri-peptide similarity and propensity. PLoS One 7:e45152. https://doi.org/10.1371/journal.pone.0045152
122. Høie MH, Gade FS, Johansen JM et al (2023) DiscoTope-3.0—improved B-cell epitope prediction using AlphaFold2 modeling and inverse folding latent representations. Front Immunol 15:1322712
123. Berman HM (2000) The Protein Data Bank. Nucleic Acids Res 28:235–242. https://doi.org/10.1093/nar/28.1.235
124. Varadi M, Anyango S, Deshpande M et al (2022) AlphaFold Protein Structure Database: massively expanding the structural coverage of protein-sequence space with high-accuracy models. Nucleic Acids Res 50:D439–D444. https://doi.org/10.1093/nar/gkab1061
125. Rubinstein ND, Mayrose I, Martz E, Pupko T (2009) Epitopia: a web-server for predicting B-cell epitopes. BMC Bioinformatics 10:287. https://doi.org/10.1186/1471-2105-10-287
126. Ansari H, Raghava GP (2010) Identification of conformational B-cell epitopes in an antigen from its primary sequence. Immunome Res 6:6. https://doi.org/10.1186/1745-7580-6-6
127. Ponomarenko J, Bui H-H, Li W et al (2008) ElliPro: a new structure-based tool for the prediction of antibody epitopes. BMC Bioinformatics 9:514. https://doi.org/10.1186/1471-2105-9-514
128. Sánchez R, Šali A (1997) Evaluation of comparative protein structure modeling by MODELLER-3. Proteins 29:50–58. https://doi.org/10.1002/(SICI)1097-0134(1997)1+<50::AID-PROT8>3.0.CO;2-S
129. Thornton JM, Edwards MS, Taylor WR, Barlow DJ (1986) Location of 'continuous' antigenic determinants in the protruding regions of proteins. EMBO J 5:409–413. https://doi.org/10.1002/j.1460-2075.1986.tb04226.x
130. Sweredoski MJ, Baldi P (2008) PEPITO: improved discontinuous B-cell epitope prediction using multiple distance thresholds and half sphere exposure. Bioinformatics 24:1459–1460. https://doi.org/10.1093/bioinformatics/btn199
131. Wang X, Fan D, Yang Y et al (2023) Integrative multi-omics approaches to explore immune cell functions: challenges and opportunities. iScience 26:106359. https://doi.org/10.1016/j.isci.2023.106359
132. Chu X, Zhang B, Koeken VACM et al (2021) Multi-omics approaches in immunological research. Front Immunol 12:668045. https://doi.org/10.3389/fimmu.2021.668045
133. Li X, Wang C-Y (2021) From bulk, single-cell to spatial RNA sequencing. Int J Oral Sci 13:36. https://doi.org/10.1038/s41368-021-00146-0
134. Saliba A-E, Westermann AJ, Gorski SA, Vogel J (2014) Single-cell RNA-seq: advances and future challenges. Nucleic Acids Res 42:8845–8860. https://doi.org/10.1093/nar/gku555
135. Hegenbarth J-C, Lezzoche G, De Windt LJ, Stoll M (2022) Perspectives on bulk-tissue RNA sequencing and single-cell RNA sequencing for cardiac transcriptomics. Front Mol Med 2:839338. https://doi.org/10.3389/fmmed.2022.839338
136. Papalexi E, Satija R (2018) Single-cell RNA sequencing to explore immune cell heterogeneity. Nat Rev Immunol 18:35–45. https://doi.org/10.1038/nri.2017.76
137. Yao C, Sun H-W, Lacey NE et al (2019) Single-cell RNA-seq reveals TOX as a key regulator of CD8+ T cell persistence in chronic infection. Nat Immunol 20:890–901. https://doi.org/10.1038/s41590-019-0403-4
138. Stewart A, Ng JC-F, Wallis G et al (2021) Single-cell transcriptomic analyses define distinct peripheral B cell subsets and discrete development pathways. Front Immunol 12:602539. https://doi.org/10.3389/fimmu.2021.602539
139. Goldstein LD, Chen Y-JJ, Wu J et al (2019) Massively parallel single-cell B-cell receptor sequencing enables rapid discovery of diverse antigen-reactive antibodies. Commun Biol 2:304. https://doi.org/10.1038/s42003-019-0551-y

140. Zemmour D, Zilionis R, Kiner E et al (2018) Single-cell gene expression reveals a landscape of regulatory T cell phenotypes shaped by the TCR. Nat Immunol 19:291–301. https://doi.org/10.1038/s41590-018-0051-0
141. Nakamura T, Yabuta Y, Okamoto I et al (2015) SC3-seq: a method for highly parallel and quantitative measurement of single-cell gene expression. Nucleic Acids Res 43:e60. https://doi.org/10.1093/nar/gkv134
142. He H, Li Z, Lu J et al (2022) Single-cell RNA-seq reveals clonal diversity and prognostic genes of relapsed multiple myeloma. Clin Transl Med 12:e757. https://doi.org/10.1002/ctm2.757
143. Gross A, Schoendube J, Zimmermann S et al (2015) Technologies for single-cell isolation. Int J Mol Sci 16:16897–16919. https://doi.org/10.3390/ijms160816897
144. Hwang B, Lee JH, Bang D (2018) Single-cell RNA sequencing technologies and bioinformatics pipelines. Exp Mol Med 50:1–14. https://doi.org/10.1038/s12276-018-0071-8
145. Tang F, Barbacioru C, Wang Y et al (2009) mRNA-Seq whole-transcriptome analysis of a single cell. Nat Methods 6:377–382. https://doi.org/10.1038/nmeth.1315
146. Sasagawa Y, Nikaido I, Hayashi T et al (2013) Quartz-Seq: a highly reproducible and sensitive single-cell RNA sequencing method, reveals non-genetic gene-expression heterogeneity. Genome Biol 14:3097. https://doi.org/10.1186/gb-2013-14-4-r31
147. Macosko EZ, Basu A, Satija R et al (2015) Highly parallel genome-wide expression profiling of individual cells using nanoliter droplets. Cell 161:1202–1214. https://doi.org/10.1016/j.cell.2015.05.002
148. Single-Cell Sequencing (2023). https://app.biorender.com/biorender-templates/figures/all/t5f2350bba193ae00b486136b-single-cell-sequencing
149. Kim D, Chung KB, Kim T-G (2020) Application of single-cell RNA sequencing on human skin: technical evolution and challenges. J Dermatol Sci 99:74–81. https://doi.org/10.1016/j.jdermsci.2020.06.002
150. Kim D, Pertea G, Trapnell C et al (2013) TopHat2: accurate alignment of transcriptomes in the presence of insertions, deletions and gene fusions. Genome Biol 14:R36. https://doi.org/10.1186/gb-2013-14-4-r36
151. Dobin A, Gingeras TR (2015) Mapping RNA-seq reads with STAR. CP Bioinformatics 51:11.14.1. https://doi.org/10.1002/0471250953.bi1114s51
152. Kim D, Langmead B, Salzberg SL (2015) HISAT: a fast spliced aligner with low memory requirements. Nat Methods 12:357–360. https://doi.org/10.1038/nmeth.3317
153. Li H, Homer N (2010) A survey of sequence alignment algorithms for next-generation sequencing. Brief Bioinformatics 11:473–483. https://doi.org/10.1093/bib/bbq015
154. Li H, Durbin R (2009) Fast and accurate short read alignment with Burrows–Wheeler transform. Bioinformatics 25:1754–1760. https://doi.org/10.1093/bioinformatics/btp324
155. Picelli S, Faridani OR, Björklund ÅK et al (2014) Full-length RNA-seq from single cells using Smart-seq2. Nat Protoc 9:171–181. https://doi.org/10.1038/nprot.2014.006
156. Sheng K, Cao W, Niu Y et al (2017) Effective detection of variation in single-cell transcriptomes using MATQ-seq. Nat Methods 14:267–270. https://doi.org/10.1038/nmeth.4145
157. Trapnell C, Williams BA, Pertea G et al (2010) Transcript assembly and quantification by RNA-Seq reveals unannotated transcripts and isoform switching during cell differentiation. Nat Biotechnol 28:511–515. https://doi.org/10.1038/nbt.1621
158. Li B, Dewey CN (2011) RSEM: accurate transcript quantification from RNA-Seq data with or without a reference genome. BMC Bioinformatics 12:323. https://doi.org/10.1186/1471-2105-12-323
159. Pertea M, Pertea GM, Antonescu CM et al (2015) StringTie enables improved reconstruction of a transcriptome from RNA-seq reads. Nat Biotechnol 33:290–295. https://doi.org/10.1038/nbt.3122
160. Glaus P, Honkela A, Rattray M (2012) Identifying differentially expressed transcripts from RNA-seq data with biological variation. Bioinformatics 28:1721–1728. https://doi.org/10.1093/bioinformatics/bts260

161. Huang M, Wang J, Torre E et al (2018) SAVER: gene expression recovery for single-cell RNA sequencing. Nat Methods 15:539–542. https://doi.org/10.1038/s41592-018-0033-z
162. Chen L, Zheng S (2018) BCseq: accurate single cell RNA-seq quantification with bias correction. Nucleic Acids Res 46:e82. https://doi.org/10.1093/nar/gky308
163. Jiang P, Thomson JA, Stewart R (2016) Quality control of single-cell RNA-seq by SinQC. Bioinformatics 32:2514–2516. https://doi.org/10.1093/bioinformatics/btw176
164. McCarthy DJ, Campbell KR, Lun ATL, Wills QF (2017) Scater: pre-processing, quality control, normalization and visualization of single-cell RNA-seq data in R. Bioinformatics 33:1179–1186. https://doi.org/10.1093/bioinformatics/btw777
165. Chidananda Gowda K, Krishna G (1978) Agglomerative clustering using the concept of mutual nearest neighbourhood. Pattern Recogn 10:105–112. https://doi.org/10.1016/0031-3203(78)90018-3
166. Büttner M, Miao Z, Wolf FA et al (2019) A test metric for assessing single-cell RNA-seq batch correction. Nat Methods 16:43–49. https://doi.org/10.1038/s41592-018-0254-1
167. Haghverdi L, Lun ATL, Morgan MD, Marioni JC (2018) Batch effects in single-cell RNA-sequencing data are corrected by matching mutual nearest neighbors. Nat Biotechnol 36:421–427. https://doi.org/10.1038/nbt.4091
168. Bacher R, Chu L-F, Leng N et al (2017) SCnorm: robust normalization of single-cell RNA-seq data. Nat Methods 14:584–586. https://doi.org/10.1038/nmeth.4263
169. Katayama S, Töhönen V, Linnarsson S, Kere J (2013) SAMstrt: statistical test for differential expression in single-cell transcriptome with spike-in normalization. Bioinformatics 29:2943–2945. https://doi.org/10.1093/bioinformatics/btt511
170. Lun ATL, Bach K, Marioni JC (2016) Pooling across cells to normalize single-cell RNA sequencing data with many zero counts. Genome Biol 17:75. https://doi.org/10.1186/s13059-016-0947-7
171. Van Dijk D, Sharma R, Nainys J et al (2018) Recovering gene interactions from single-cell data using data diffusion. Cell 174:716–729.e27. https://doi.org/10.1016/j.cell.2018.05.061
172. Hafemeister C, Satija R (2019) Normalization and variance stabilization of single-cell RNA-seq data using regularized negative binomial regression. Genome Biol 20:296. https://doi.org/10.1186/s13059-019-1874-1
173. Belkina AC, Ciccolella CO, Anno R et al (2019) Automated optimized parameters for T-distributed stochastic neighbor embedding improve visualization and analysis of large datasets. Nat Commun 10:5415. https://doi.org/10.1038/s41467-019-13055-y
174. Wold S, Esbensen K, Geladi P (1987) Principal component analysis. Chemom Intell Lab Syst 2:37–52. https://doi.org/10.1016/0169-7439(87)80084-9
175. McInnes L, Healy J, Melville J (2018) UMAP: uniform manifold approximation and projection for dimension reduction. https://doi.org/10.48550/ARXIV.1802.03426
176. Blondel VD, Guillaume J-L, Lambiotte R, Lefebvre E (2008) Fast unfolding of communities in large networks. https://doi.org/10.48550/ARXIV.0803.0476
177. Kriegel H, Kröger P, Sander J, Zimek A (2011) Density-based clustering. WIREs Data Min Knowl 1:231–240. https://doi.org/10.1002/widm.30
178. Žurauskienė J, Yau C (2016) pcaReduce: hierarchical clustering of single cell transcriptional profiles. BMC Bioinformatics 17:140. https://doi.org/10.1186/s12859-016-0984-y
179. Likas A, Vlassis N, Verbeek JJ (2003) The global k-means clustering algorithm. Pattern Recogn 36:451–461. https://doi.org/10.1016/S0031-3203(02)00060-2
180. Kiselev VY, Kirschner K, Schaub MT et al (2017) SC3: consensus clustering of single-cell RNA-seq data. Nat Methods 14:483–486. https://doi.org/10.1038/nmeth.4236
181. Hao Y, Stuart T, Kowalski MH et al (2024) Dictionary learning for integrative, multimodal and scalable single-cell analysis. Nat Biotechnol 42:293–304. https://doi.org/10.1038/s41587-023-01767-y
182. Love MI, Huber W, Anders S (2014) Moderated estimation of fold change and dispersion for RNA-seq data with DESeq2. Genome Biol 15:550. https://doi.org/10.1186/s13059-014-0550-8

183. Finak G, McDavid A, Yajima M et al (2015) MAST: a flexible statistical framework for assessing transcriptional changes and characterizing heterogeneity in single-cell RNA sequencing data. Genome Biol 16:278. https://doi.org/10.1186/s13059-015-0844-5
184. Kharchenko PV, Silberstein L, Scadden DT (2014) Bayesian approach to single-cell differential expression analysis. Nat Methods 11:740–742. https://doi.org/10.1038/nmeth.2967
185. Miao Z, Deng K, Wang X, Zhang X (2018) DEsingle for detecting three types of differential expression in single-cell RNA-seq data. Bioinformatics 34:3223–3224. https://doi.org/10.1093/bioinformatics/bty332
186. Qiu X, Hill A, Packer J et al (2017) Single-cell mRNA quantification and differential analysis with Census. Nat Methods 14:309–315. https://doi.org/10.1038/nmeth.4150
187. Mao G, Pang Z, Zuo K et al (2023) Predicting gene regulatory links from single-cell RNA-seq data using graph neural networks. Brief Bioinform 24:bbad414. https://doi.org/10.1093/bib/bbad414
188. Chan TE, Stumpf MPH, Babtie AC (2017) Gene regulatory network inference from single-cell data using multivariate information measures. Cell Syst 5:251–267.e3. https://doi.org/10.1016/j.cels.2017.08.014
189. Nathan A, Baglaenko Y, Fonseka CY et al (2019) Multimodal single-cell approaches shed light on T cell heterogeneity. Curr Opin Immunol 61:17–25. https://doi.org/10.1016/j.coi.2019.07.002
190. Stubbington MJT, Lönnberg T, Proserpio V et al (2016) T cell fate and clonality inference from single-cell transcriptomes. Nat Methods 13:329–332. https://doi.org/10.1038/nmeth.3800
191. Matsumoto H, Kiryu H, Furusawa C et al (2017) SCODE: an efficient regulatory network inference algorithm from single-cell RNA-Seq during differentiation. Bioinformatics 33:2314–2321. https://doi.org/10.1093/bioinformatics/btx194
192. Ginsburg GS, Willard HF (2010) Essentials of genomic and personalized medicine. Elsevier, Amsterdam
193. Dettmer K, Aronov PA, Hammock BD (2007) Mass spectrometry-based metabolomics. Mass Spectrom Rev 26:51–78. https://doi.org/10.1002/mas.20108
194. Samuelsson J, Dalevi D, Levander F, Rögnvaldsson T (2004) Modular, scriptable and automated analysis tools for high-throughput peptide mass fingerprinting. Bioinformatics 20:3628–3635. https://doi.org/10.1093/bioinformatics/bth460
195. Fenn JB, Mann M, Meng CK et al (1989) Electrospray ionization for mass spectrometry of large biomolecules. Science 246:64–71. https://doi.org/10.1126/science.2675315
196. Aiken AC, DeCarlo PF, Jimenez JL (2007) Elemental analysis of organic species with electron ionization high-resolution mass spectrometry. Anal Chem 79:8350–8358. https://doi.org/10.1021/ac071150w
197. Hillenkamp F, Karas M, Beavis RC, Chait BT (1991) Matrix-assisted laser desorption/ionization mass spectrometry of biopolymers. Anal Chem 63:1193A–1203A. https://doi.org/10.1021/ac00024a716
198. Andrade FJ, Shelley JT, Wetzel WC et al (2008) Atmospheric pressure chemical ionization source. 1. Ionization of compounds in the gas phase. Anal Chem 80:2646–2653. https://doi.org/10.1021/ac800156y
199. Smith R, Mathis AD, Ventura D, Prince JT (2014) Proteomics, lipidomics, metabolomics: a mass spectrometry tutorial from a computer scientist's point of view. BMC Bioinformatics 15:S9. https://doi.org/10.1186/1471-2105-15-S7-S9
200. Niessen WMA (1999) Liquid chromatography—mass spectrometry, 2nd ed., rev. expanded edn. M. Dekker, New York
201. Garcia A, Barbas C (2011) Gas chromatography-mass spectrometry (GC-MS)-based metabolomics. In: Metz TO (ed) Metabolic profiling. Humana, Totowa, NJ, pp 191–204
202. Mischak H, Coon JJ, Novak J et al (2009) Capillary electrophoresis–mass spectrometry as a powerful tool in biomarker discovery and clinical diagnosis: an update of recent developments. Mass Spectrom Rev 28:703–724. https://doi.org/10.1002/mas.20205
203. Rew R, Davis G, Emmerson S et al (1989) Unidata NetCDF

204. Pedrioli PGA, Eng JK, Hubley R et al (2004) A common open representation of mass spectrometry data and its application to proteomics research. Nat Biotechnol 22:1459–1466. https://doi.org/10.1038/nbt1031
205. Kurgaev AF, Grigoriev SN (2017) Definition of the languages XML and RDF of the semantic web in the metalanguage of normal forms of knowledge. Cybern Syst Anal 53:684–691. https://doi.org/10.1007/s10559-017-9970-2
206. Brusniak M-Y, Bodenmiller B, Campbell D et al (2008) Corra: computational framework and tools for LC-MS discovery and targeted mass spectrometry-based proteomics. BMC Bioinformatics 9:542. https://doi.org/10.1186/1471-2105-9-542
207. Teo GC, Polasky DA, Yu F, Nesvizhskii AI (2021) Fast deisotoping algorithm and its implementation in the MSFragger search engine. J Proteome Res 20:498–505. https://doi.org/10.1021/acs.jproteome.0c00544
208. Fahy E, Subramaniam S, Murphy RC et al (2009) Update of the LIPID MAPS comprehensive classification system for lipids. J Lipid Res 50:S9–S14. https://doi.org/10.1194/jlr.R800095-JLR200
209. Smith CA, Maille GO, Want EJ et al (2005) METLIN: a metabolite mass spectral database. Ther Drug Monit 27:747–751. https://doi.org/10.1097/01.ftd.0000179845.53213.39
210. Thomas T, Gilbert J, Meyer F (2012) Metagenomics—a guide from sampling to data analysis. Microb Informatics Exp 2:3. https://doi.org/10.1186/2042-5783-2-3
211. Tang W, Zhang Y, Luo C et al (2021) Clinical application of metagenomic next-generation sequencing for suspected infections in patients with primary immunodeficiency disease. Front Immunol 12:696403. https://doi.org/10.3389/fimmu.2021.696403
212. Al-Nesf MA, Morgan D, Mohamed-Ali V (2021) Primary immunodeficiency and the microbiome. Curr Opin Pediatr 33:633–638. https://doi.org/10.1097/MOP.0000000000001067
213. Salipante SJ, Sengupta DJ, Rosenthal C et al (2013) Rapid 16S rRNA next-generation sequencing of polymicrobial clinical samples for diagnosis of complex bacterial infections. PLoS One 8:e65226. https://doi.org/10.1371/journal.pone.0065226
214. Chiu CY, Miller SA (2019) Clinical metagenomics. Nat Rev Genet 20:341–355. https://doi.org/10.1038/s41576-019-0113-7
215. García-García G, Baux D, Faugère V et al (2016) Assessment of the latest NGS enrichment capture methods in clinical context. Sci Rep 6:20948. https://doi.org/10.1038/srep20948
216. Castañeda-Mogollón D, Kamaliddin C, Oberding L et al (2021) A metagenomics workflow for SARS-CoV-2 identification, co-pathogen detection, and overall diversity. J Clin Virol 145:105025. https://doi.org/10.1016/j.jcv.2021.105025
217. Dash HR, Das S (2018) Molecular methods for studying microorganisms from atypical environments, Methods in microbiology. Elsevier, pp 89–122
218. Rifai N, Gillette MA, Carr SA (2006) Protein biomarker discovery and validation: the long and uncertain path to clinical utility. Nat Biotechnol 24:971–983. https://doi.org/10.1038/nbt1235
219. Park J, Munagala I, Xu H et al (2013) Interferon signature in the blood in inflammatory common variable immune deficiency. PLoS One 8:e74893. https://doi.org/10.1371/journal.pone.0074893
220. Warnatz K, Denz A, Dräger R et al (2002) Severe deficiency of switched memory B cells (CD27+IgM−IgD−) in subgroups of patients with common variable immunodeficiency: a new approach to classify a heterogeneous disease. Blood 99:1544–1551. https://doi.org/10.1182/blood.V99.5.1544
221. Wehr C, Kivioja T, Schmitt C et al (2008) The EUROclass trial: defining subgroups in common variable immunodeficiency. Blood 111:77–85. https://doi.org/10.1182/blood-2007-06-091744
222. Malphettes M, Gérard L, Carmagnat M et al (2009) Late-onset combined immune deficiency: a subset of common variable immunodeficiency with severe T cell defect. Clin Infect Dis 49:1329–1338. https://doi.org/10.1086/606059
223. Azizi G, Abolhassani H, Kiaee F et al (2018) Autoimmunity and its association with regulatory T cells and B cell subsets in patients with common variable immunodeficiency. Allergol Immunopathol 46:127–135. https://doi.org/10.1016/j.aller.2017.04.004

224. Melo KM, Carvalho KI, Bruno FR et al (2009) A decreased frequency of regulatory T cells in patients with common variable immunodeficiency. PLoS One 4:e6269. https://doi.org/10.1371/journal.pone.0006269
225. Horn J, Manguiat A, Berglund LJ et al (2009) Decrease in phenotypic regulatory T cells in subsets of patients with common variable immunodeficiency. Clin Exp Immunol 156:446–454. https://doi.org/10.1111/j.1365-2249.2009.03913.x
226. Nehme NT, Schmid JP, Debeurme F et al (2012) MST1 mutations in autosomal recessive primary immunodeficiency characterized by defective naive T-cell survival. Blood 119:3458–3468. https://doi.org/10.1182/blood-2011-09-378364
227. North ME, Webster ADB, Farrant J (2001) Primary defect in CD8+ lymphocytes in the antibody deficiency disease (common variable immunodeficiency): abnormalities in intracellular production of interferon-gamma (IFN-γ) in CD28+ ('cytotoxic') and CD28− ('suppressor') CD8+ subsets. Clin Exp Immunol 111:70–75. https://doi.org/10.1046/j.1365-2249.1998.00479.x
228. Varzaneh FN, Keller B, Unger S et al (2014) Cytokines in common variable immunodeficiency as signs of immune dysregulation and potential therapeutic targets—a review of the current knowledge. J Clin Immunol 34:524–543. https://doi.org/10.1007/s10875-014-0053-0
229. Unger S, Seidl M, Van Schouwenburg P et al (2018) The TH1 phenotype of follicular helper T cells indicates an IFN-γ–associated immune dysregulation in patients with CD21low common variable immunodeficiency. J Allergy Clin Immunol 141:730–740. https://doi.org/10.1016/j.jaci.2017.04.041
230. Cols M, Rahman A, Maglione PJ et al (2016) Expansion of inflammatory innate lymphoid cells in patients with common variable immune deficiency. J Allergy Clin Immunol 137:1206–1215.e6. https://doi.org/10.1016/j.jaci.2015.09.013
231. Ho H, Radigan L, Bongers G et al (2021) Circulating bioactive bacterial DNA is associated with immune activation and complications in common variable immunodeficiency. JCI Insight 6:e144777. https://doi.org/10.1172/jci.insight.144777
232. Eisenstein EM, Jaffe JS, Strober W (1993) Reduced interleukin-2 (IL-2) production in common variable immunodeficiency is due to a primary abnormality of CD4+ T cell differentiation. J Clin Immunol 13:247–258. https://doi.org/10.1007/BF00919383
233. Knight AK, Radigan L, Marron T et al (2007) High serum levels of BAFF, APRIL, and TACI in common variable immunodeficiency. Clin Immunol 124:182–189. https://doi.org/10.1016/j.clim.2007.04.012
234. Maglione PJ, Ko HM, Tokuyama M et al (2020) Serum B-cell maturation antigen (BCMA) levels differentiate primary antibody deficiencies. J Allergy Clin Immunol Pract 8:283–291.e1. https://doi.org/10.1016/j.jaip.2019.08.012
235. Chapel H, Lucas M, Lee M et al (2008) Common variable immunodeficiency disorders: division into distinct clinical phenotypes. Blood 112:277–286. https://doi.org/10.1182/blood-2007-11-124545
236. Macpherson ME, Halvorsen B, Yndestad A et al (2019) Impaired HDL function amplifies systemic inflammation in common variable immunodeficiency. Sci Rep 9:9427. https://doi.org/10.1038/s41598-019-45861-1
237. Barbosa RR, Silva SP, Silva SL et al (2012) Monocyte activation is a feature of common variable immunodeficiency irrespective of plasma lipopolysaccharide levels. Clin Exp Immunol 169:263–272. https://doi.org/10.1111/j.1365-2249.2012.04620.x
238. Litzman J, Nechvatalova J, Xu J et al (2012) Chronic immune activation in common variable immunodeficiency (CVID) is associated with elevated serum levels of soluble CD14 and CD25 but not endotoxaemia. Clin Exp Immunol 170:321–332. https://doi.org/10.1111/j.1365-2249.2012.04655.x
239. Schaid DJ, Rowland CM, Tines DE et al (2002) Score tests for association between traits and haplotypes when linkage phase is ambiguous. Am J Hum Genet 70:425–434. https://doi.org/10.1086/338688
240. Sanchez-Mazas A, Vidan-Jeras B, Nunes JM et al (2012) Strategies to work with HLA data in human populations for histocompatibility, clinical transplantation, epidemiology and popula-

tion genetics: HLA-NET methodological recommendations. Int J Immunogenet 39:459–476. https://doi.org/10.1111/j.1744-313X.2012.01113.x
241. Boegel S, Löwer M, Schäfer M et al (2012) HLA typing from RNA-Seq sequence reads. Genome Med 4:102. https://doi.org/10.1186/gm403
242. Castagnoli R, Delmonte OM, Calzoni E, Notarangelo LD (2019) Hematopoietic stem cell transplantation in primary immunodeficiency diseases: current status and future perspectives. Front Pediatr 7:295. https://doi.org/10.3389/fped.2019.00295
243. Urban C, Schmidt AH, Hofmann JA (2020) Hap-E search 2.0: improving the performance of a probabilistic donor-recipient matching algorithm based on haplotype frequencies. Front Med 7:32. https://doi.org/10.3389/fmed.2020.00032
244. Bochtler W, Eberhard H-P, Beth M, Mueller CR (2008) 136: Optimatch®—optimized selection of allele matched unrelated donors from a large database. Biol Blood Marrow Transplant 14:52. https://doi.org/10.1016/j.bbmt.2007.12.145
245. Dubois V, Detrait M, Sobh M et al (2016) Using EasyMatch® to anticipate the identification of an HLA identical unrelated donor: a validated efficient time and cost saving method. Hum Immunol 77:1008–1015. https://doi.org/10.1016/j.humimm.2016.02.004
246. Dehn J, Setterholm M, Buck K et al (2016) HapLogic: a predictive human leukocyte antigen–matching algorithm to enhance rapid identification of the optimal unrelated hematopoietic stem cell sources for transplantation. Biol Blood Marrow Transplant 22:2038–2046. https://doi.org/10.1016/j.bbmt.2016.07.022
247. Sinnwell JP, Schaid DJ (2024) Package Haplo.Stats: statistical analysis of haplotypes with traits and covariates when linkage phase is ambiguous
248. Kohn LA, Kohn DB (2021) Gene therapies for primary immune deficiencies. Front Immunol 12:648951. https://doi.org/10.3389/fimmu.2021.648951
249. Schwarzer A, Talbot SR, Selich A et al (2021) Predicting genotoxicity of viral vectors for stem cell gene therapy using gene expression-based machine learning. Mol Ther 29:3383–3397. https://doi.org/10.1016/j.ymthe.2021.06.017
250. Wessels H-H, Stirn A, Méndez-Mancilla A et al (2023) Prediction of on-target and off-target activity of CRISPR–Cas13d guide RNAs using deep learning. Nat Biotechnol 42:628. https://doi.org/10.1038/s41587-023-01830-8
251. Chavda V, Anand K, Apostolopoulos V (2023) Bioinformatics tools for pharmaceutical drug product development, 1st edn. Wiley
252. Yang F, Zhang Q, Ji X et al (2022) Machine learning applications in drug repurposing. Interdiscip Sci Comput Life Sci 14:15–21. https://doi.org/10.1007/s12539-021-00487-8
253. Wang P, Liu C, Wei Z et al (2023) Nomogram for predicting early mortality after umbilical cord blood transplantation in children with inborn errors of immunity. J Clin Immunol 43:1379–1392. https://doi.org/10.1007/s10875-023-01505-8
254. Andronis C, Sharma A, Virvilis V et al (2011) Literature mining, ontologies and information visualization for drug repurposing. Brief Bioinform 12:357–368. https://doi.org/10.1093/bib/bbr005
255. Hosmer DW, Lemeshow S, Sturdivant RX (2013) Applied logistic regression, 1st edn. Wiley
256. Huang K, Fu T, Glass LM et al (2021) DeepPurpose: a deep learning library for drug–target interaction prediction. Bioinformatics 36:5545–5547. https://doi.org/10.1093/bioinformatics/btaa1005
257. Cheng J, Dong L, Lapata M (2016) Long short-term memory-networks for machine Reading. https://doi.org/10.48550/ARXIV.1601.06733
258. Volkamer A, Kuhn D, Rippmann F, Rarey M (2012) DoGSiteScorer: a web server for automatic binding site prediction, analysis and druggability assessment. Bioinformatics 28:2074–2075. https://doi.org/10.1093/bioinformatics/bts310
259. Hajduk PJ, Huth JR, Tse C (2005) Predicting protein druggability. Drug Discov Today 10:1675–1682. https://doi.org/10.1016/S1359-6446(05)03624-X
260. Garcia-Perez L, Van Eggermond M, Van Roon L et al (2020) Successful preclinical development of gene therapy for recombinase-activating gene-1-deficient SCID. Mol Ther Methods Clin Dev 17:666–682. https://doi.org/10.1016/j.omtm.2020.03.016

261. Valencic E, Grasso AG, Conversano E et al (2018) Theophylline as a precision therapy in a young girl with PIK3R1 immunodeficiency. J Allergy Clin Immunol Pract 6:2165–2167. https://doi.org/10.1016/j.jaip.2018.02.029
262. Van Coillie S, Wiernicki B, Xu J (2020) Molecular and cellular functions of CTLA-4. In: Xu J (ed) Regulation of cancer immune checkpoints. Springer Singapore, Singapore, pp 7–32
263. Lopez-Herrera G, Tampella G, Pan-Hammarström Q et al (2012) Deleterious mutations in LRBA are associated with a syndrome of immune deficiency and autoimmunity. Am J Hum Genet 90:986–1001. https://doi.org/10.1016/j.ajhg.2012.04.015
264. Charbonnier L-M, Janssen E, Chou J et al (2015) Regulatory T-cell deficiency and immune dysregulation, polyendocrinopathy, enteropathy, X-linked–like disorder caused by loss-of-function mutations in LRBA. J Allergy Clin Immunol 135:217–227.e9. https://doi.org/10.1016/j.jaci.2014.10.019
265. Gámez-Díaz L, August D, Stepensky P et al (2016) The extended phenotype of LPS-responsive beige-like anchor protein (LRBA) deficiency. J Allergy Clin Immunol 137:223–230. https://doi.org/10.1016/j.jaci.2015.09.025
266. Schwab C, Gabrysch A, Olbrich P et al (2018) Phenotype, penetrance, and treatment of 133 cytotoxic T-lymphocyte antigen 4–insufficient subjects. J Allergy Clin Immunol 142:1932–1946. https://doi.org/10.1016/j.jaci.2018.02.055
267. Lee S, Moon JS, Lee C-R et al (2016) Abatacept alleviates severe autoimmune symptoms in a patient carrying a de novo variant in CTLA-4. J Allergy Clin Immunol 137:327–330. https://doi.org/10.1016/j.jaci.2015.08.036
268. Lye JJ, Williams A, Baralle D (2019) Exploring the RNA gap for improving diagnostic yield in primary immunodeficiencies. Front Genet 10:1204. https://doi.org/10.3389/fgene.2019.01204
269. Sheikh H, Prins C, Schrijvers E (2023) Artificial intelligence: definition and background. In: Mission AI. Springer International Publishing, Cham, pp 15–41
270. Rider NL, Srinivasan R, Khoury P (2020) Artificial intelligence and the hunt for immunological disorders. Curr Opin Allergy Clin Immunol 20:565–573. https://doi.org/10.1097/ACI.0000000000000691
271. Sarker IH (2021) Machine learning: algorithms, real-world applications and research directions. SN Comput Sci 2:160. https://doi.org/10.1007/s42979-021-00592-x
272. Charbuty B, Abdulazeez A (2021) Classification based on decision tree algorithm for machine learning. J Appl Sci Technol Trends 2:20–28. https://doi.org/10.38094/jastt20165
273. Hearst MA, Dumais ST, Osuna E et al (1998) Support vector machines. IEEE Intell Syst Appl 13:18–28. https://doi.org/10.1109/5254.708428
274. Keller JM, Gray MR, Givens JA (1985) A fuzzy K-nearest neighbor algorithm. IEEE Trans Syst Man Cybernet SMC-15:580–585. https://doi.org/10.1109/TSMC.1985.6313426
275. Webb GI (2011) Naïve Bayes. In: Sammut C, Webb GI (eds) Encyclopedia of machine learning. Springer, Boston, MA, pp 713–714
276. Modell V, Quinn J, Ginsberg G et al (2017) Modeling strategy to identify patients with primary immunodeficiency utilizing risk management and outcome measurement. Immunol Res 65:713–720. https://doi.org/10.1007/s12026-017-8907-1
277. Rider NL, Miao D, Dodds M et al (2019) Calculation of a primary immunodeficiency "risk vital sign" via population-wide analysis of claims data to aid in clinical decision support. Front Pediatr 7:70. https://doi.org/10.3389/fped.2019.00070
278. Mayampurath A, Ajith A, Anderson-Smits C et al (2022) Early diagnosis of primary immunodeficiency disease using clinical data and machine learning. J Allergy Clin Immunol Pract 10:3002–3007.e5. https://doi.org/10.1016/j.jaip.2022.08.041
279. Köhler S, Carmody L, Vasilevsky N et al (2019) Expansion of the Human Phenotype Ontology (HPO) knowledge base and resources. Nucleic Acids Res 47:D1018–D1027. https://doi.org/10.1093/nar/gky1105
280. Zhang XA, Yates A, Vasilevsky N et al (2019) Semantic integration of clinical laboratory tests from electronic health records for deep phenotyping and biomarker discovery. npj Digit Med 2:32. https://doi.org/10.1038/s41746-019-0110-4

281. Norori N, Hu Q, Aellen FM et al (2021) Addressing bias in big data and AI for health care: a call for open science. Patterns 2:100347. https://doi.org/10.1016/j.patter.2021.100347
282. Mackay TF, Moore JH (2014) Why epistasis is important for tackling complex human disease genetics. Genome Med 6:42. https://doi.org/10.1186/gm561
283. Woodward AA, Urbanowicz RJ, Naj AC, Moore JH (2022) Genetic heterogeneity: challenges, impacts, and methods through an associative lens. Genet Epidemiol 46:555–571. https://doi.org/10.1002/gepi.22497
284. Nussinov R, Tsai C-J, Shehu A, Jang H (2019) Computational structural biology: successes, future directions, and challenges. Molecules 24:637. https://doi.org/10.3390/molecules24030637
285. Varadi M, Bertoni D, Magana P et al (2024) AlphaFold Protein Structure Database in 2024: providing structure coverage for over 214 million protein sequences. Nucleic Acids Res 52:D368–D375. https://doi.org/10.1093/nar/gkad1011
286. Decherchi S, Pedrini E, Mordenti M et al (2021) Opportunities and challenges for machine learning in rare diseases. Front Med 8:747612. https://doi.org/10.3389/fmed.2021.747612

Clinical Management of Severe Combined Immunodeficiencies

4

Francesco Pegoraro, Marta Voarino,
and Eleonora Gambineri

4.1 Introduction

Severe combined immunodeficiency (SCID) includes several inherited disorders of T- and B-lymphocyte function that make affected individuals severely susceptible to infections, making early diagnosis and prompt management critical for survival. This requires a multidisciplinary approach in order to address the many criticalities of these conditions [1]. The curative treatment for SCID is hematopoietic stem cell transplantation (HSCT), which restores the immune system; however, this strategy must be implemented as soon as possible, together with antimicrobial prophylaxis and supportive measures to bridge the patient to HSCT in the best clinical condition [1, 2]. The effectiveness of this management strategy, aiming to perform HSCT before serious infectious complications, is greatly improved by newborn screening. Gene therapy is an alternative approach to HSCT, which is limited to specific genetic mutations (mostly adenosine deaminase deficiency) and has its own criticalities [3].

F. Pegoraro
Department of Experimental and Clinical Medicine, University of Florence, Florence, Italy

Department of Hematology and Oncology, Meyer Children's Hospital IRCCS, Florence, Italy

M. Voarino
Department of Health Sciences, University of Florence, Florence, Italy

E. Gambineri (✉)
Department of Hematology and Oncology, Meyer Children's Hospital IRCCS, Florence, Italy

Department of Neurosciences, Psychology, Drug Research and Child Health (NEUROFARBA), University of Florence, Florence, Italy
e-mail: eleonora.gambineri@unifi.it

M. M. D'Elios (ed.), *Severe Combined Immunodeficiency*, Rare Diseases of the Immune System, https://doi.org/10.1007/978-3-031-78864-2_4

4.2 General Management

Patients with a suspected or confirmed diagnosis of SCID require a multidisciplinary management approach in order to bridge them to the potentially corrective procedure in the best possible condition. In the first instance, protective strategies must be put in place to prevent infection; these strategies include antimicrobial prophylaxis and isolation measures, even before the diagnosis is confirmed. Once the specific defect is identified, the definitive treatment strategy should be chosen and put in motion with the least possible delay [1, 4] (Fig. 4.1).

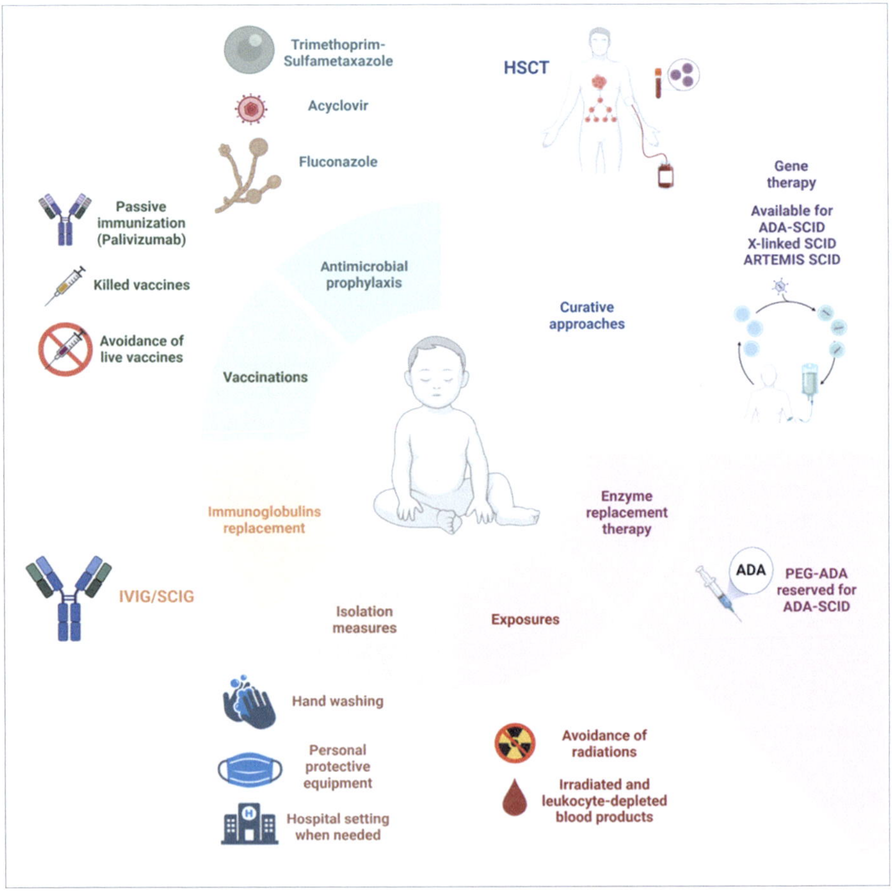

Fig. 4.1 Comprehensive management of severe combined immunodeficiencies. *IVIG* intravenous immunoglobulin, *SCIG* subcutaneous immunoglobulins, *HSCT* hematopoietic stem cells transplant, *(ADA)-SCID* adenosine deaminase deficiency, *PEG-ADA* pegylated-adenosine deaminase. (Adapted from "Nanotherapeutics in Cancer," by BioRender.com (2024). Retrieved from https://app.biorender.com/biorender-templates. Created with BioRender.com)

4.2.1 Antimicrobial Prophylaxis

4.2.1.1 *Pneumocystis jirovecii* Pneumonia

The first choice for *P. jirovecii* pneumonia prevention is oral treatment with sulfamethoxazole and trimethoprim 3 days a week, with doses adapted to the patient's weight. The most used scheme consists of 5 mg/kg (on trimethoprim) daily in two doses. The maximal daily dose in older children, adolescents, and adults is 160 mg (on trimethoprim) twice. For younger children, oral liquid formulations are available [1]. Alternative prophylactic regimens (i.e., pentamidine, dapsone, and atovaquone) are reported in Table 4.1.

4.2.1.2 Immunoglobulins for Antibody Replacement

Intravenous immune globulin (IVIG) and subcutaneous immune globulin (SCIG) are administered at a standard initial dose of 400 mg/kg (up to 600) every 3–4 weeks (IVIG) and 100–200 mg/kg weekly (SCIG). Serum IgG level should be monitored every 3–6 months, but there is no universally accepted threshold of serum IgG to indicate replacement efficacy (range between >400 and >800 mg/dL), which also depends on the clinical response in terms of infection rate. After HSCT, IgG replacement is usually required for the first 1–2 years [1, 5]. Of note, the positioning of a permanent central catheter for IVIG administration is discouraged because of the risk of infectious complications.

4.2.1.3 Others

Acyclovir can be used for HSV and VZV infection prevention, depending on the specific error of immunity or in case of suspected or confirmed exposure to the virus. In addition, palivizumab prophylaxis against respiratory syncytial virus can be proposed for patients with SCID, based on the American Academy of Pediatrics recommendations [6]. Although there is no specific indication for nirsevimab in SCID, this novel agent is likely to be progressively introduced also in this context.

Table 4.1 Regimens for Pneumocystis pneumonia prophylaxis in children and adults

	Pediatric dosing		Adults and adolescents
Trimethoprim-sulfamethoxazole	5 mg TMP/kg/day (maximum dose 160 mg TMP/dose, 320 mg TMP/day), divided in two doses and administered 3 days per week		160 mg TMP/day administered daily
Dapsone	2 mg/kg/day (maximum dose 100 mg/day)		100 mg/day, in one or two doses
Atovaquone (oral suspension)	30 mg/kg/day (maximum dose 1500 mg/day)		1500 mg/day
Pentamidine	Children <5 years of age: *intravenous* pentamidine, 4 mg/kg/dose (maximum dose 300 mg/dose), once every 4 weeks	Children >5 years of age: *aerosolized* pentamidine, 300 mg, once every 4 weeks	Aerosolized pentamidine 300 mg, once every 4 weeks

TMP trimethoprim

Antibiotic prophylaxis for respiratory tract infections other than *P. jirovecii* pneumonia prevention should be proposed based on the specific defect or in addition to Ig replacement, depending on the clinical picture [1]. Regimens for prophylaxis of bacterial respiratory tract infections include amoxicillin, azithromycin, or clarithromycin and inhaled aminoglycosides. Finally, fluconazole prophylaxis can be used for *Candida* spp. infections (6 mg/kg twice weekly, parenteral or enteral administration).

4.2.2 Exposure to Vaccines, Radiation, and Blood Products

Live vaccines are contraindicated in patients with SCID for the risk of disseminated disease in severely immunocompromised patients [1, 7]. These live vaccines include the bacille Calmette-Guerin, the oral poliovirus, the measles-mumps-rubella, the oral typhoid, the varicella, the yellow fever, and the rotavirus vaccines. Conversely, killed or microbial subcomponent vaccines can be safely administered according to routine schedules [7, 8]. Moreover, radiation exposure should be limited, especially in patients diagnosed with radiation-sensitive SCID (e.g., Artemis, DNA Ligase IV, DNA-PKcs, Cernunnos-XLF, and nibrin). Finally, when the transfusion of a blood component is required, products should be irradiated, CMV-negative, and lymphocyte-depleted. This can prevent the development of graft-versus-host disease (GVHD) and CMV opportunistic infections.

4.2.3 Isolation Measures and Other Considerations

Protection from exposure to infectious agents is crucial in patients with severe immune system deficiencies, especially for those candidates for HSCT, as the presence of severe infections significantly decreases post-HSCT survival. The management setting (hospital vs. home) should be tailored case to case, based on the social situation of the family, the presence of young children at home, the house's proximity to the hospital, and the risk of nosocomial infections. As a general rule, public or crowded places should be avoided, even in the hospital setting. In this scenario, standard isolation measures (i.e., cleaning of the room, hand washing, mask and gloves, and time planning to avoid busy waiting rooms) must be applied. Counseling of caregivers on infection prevention is also essential, and interaction with the patient must be limited to individuals with up-to-date vaccinations. Due to the potential risk of CMV transmission through breastfeeding in women with positive CMV serology, breastfeeding is generally not recommended, even though there is no definitive evidence against it.

Patients with SCID should be evaluated for potential infections such as CMV, EBV, and HIV. Moreover, prompt vigilance for infections and early empiric treatment initiation are crucial in the clinical management of patients with suspected or confirmed SCID. Of note, antimicrobial treatment is usually prolonged in patients with SCID. Finally, infants with Omenn's syndrome or maternal engraftment might require immunosuppressive treatment to reduce their intrinsic pro-inflammatory status [9].

4.3 HSCT

SCID is considered an almost inevitably fatal condition in the first decade of life unless definitive treatment is promptly administered. HSCT is the definitive treatment for SCID but is still burdened by life-threatening disease- and transplant-related complications [3]. Moreover, although outcomes of HSCT in Inborn Errors of Immunity (IEI) have significantly improved in the last decades due to better donor selection, conditioning regimens, and supportive care, the limited availability of optimal donors and the potential exposure to severe infection before HSCT still have the potential to significantly impact HSCT outcome and patient survival [3, 10].

Therefore, the age at diagnosis and the infectious status of the patient are crucial determinants of HSCT outcome [11]. Several studies have linked a younger age at HSCT (e.g., 1 month, 3.5 months) with improved survival [12, 13]. In this regard, neonatal screening plays a central role in early identification, and thus early treatment and better outcomes, of SCID [14].

Of note, replacement therapy with a pegylated enzyme is available for patients with ADA-SCID. This allows an even partial improvement of lymphocyte fitness via the removal of excess purine intermediates and makes HSCT less urgent for these patients [15].

4.3.1 Type of Donor

HLA-matched related donors (MRD) are the first choice in patients with SCID, with survival rates reaching 90% in recent years [14, 16]. The use of an MRD is associated with better overall and graft survival. Therefore, right after SCID diagnosis, HLA typing should be promptly performed on family members. Bone marrow should be used as the stem cell source.

Alternatively, a matched unrelated donor can be used. Survival is reported to be similar or just slightly inferior, compared to HSCT using an MRD [17, 18]. However, this strategy implies a longer delay from the diagnosis to the graft, due to the time needed for donor selection, and this can result in a major infectious burden before transplant. A haploidentical parent, a mismatched related donor, or a cord blood donor can be also used. The survival after haploidentical HSCT has greatly improved in the last decades (~90%) and is getting close to that of MRD [12, 16, 19]. T-cell depletion strategies, both in vivo and ex vivo, are used to reduce the rate of GVHD. Finally, the use of cord blood-derived stem cells has been associated with contrasting results and might be associated with inferior survival [11, 20], probably since infused T cells are functionally naive and post-transplantation immune reconstitution is slower. In any case, this graft source should be used when the center has great expertise in this strategy [21] (Fig. 4.2)

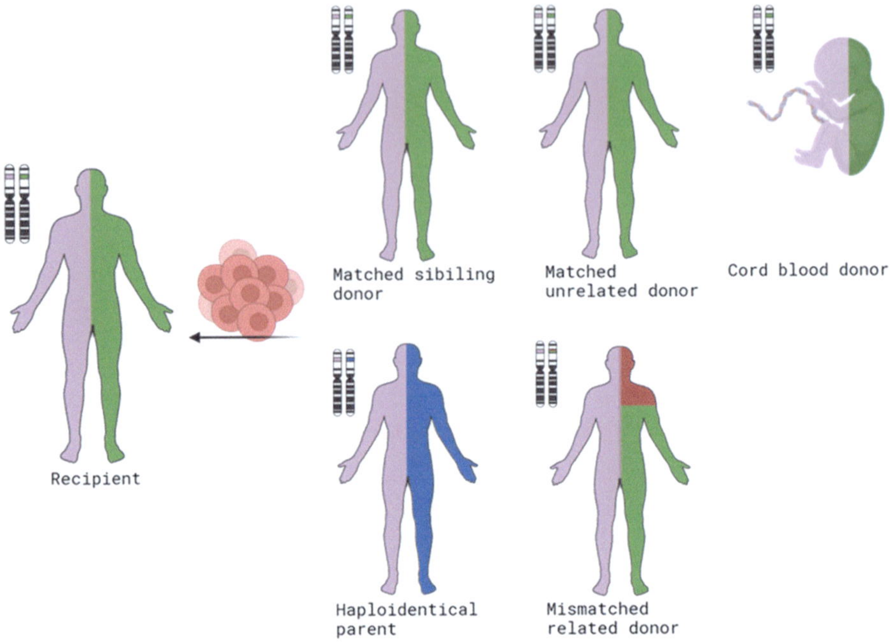

Fig. 4.2 Potential hematopoietic stem cell donors categorized by degree of HLA matching. (Created with BioRender.com)

4.3.2 Conditioning

The intrinsic nature of SCID has significant implications concerning conditioning. In many genetic defects causing SCID, the resistance to grafted stem cells is minimal or even absent, and therefore the use of conditioning could be avoided [4]. In a recent large study on 338 SCID patients, no difference in overall survival was found between patients who received conditioning and those who did not [10]. However, in the latest ESID/EBMT guidelines, conditioning was recommended for all types of SCID [2]. Immunoablative (fludarabine, cyclophosphamide, ATG, alemtuzumab) or myeloablative (melphalan, treosulfan, busulfan) conditioning regimens can be used [2]. When a myeloablative regimen is proposed, choosing reduced-intensity conditioning (RIC), by reducing busulfan dose (50–60%) or treosulfan, can reduce toxicity and improve survival [2, 22, 23]. Myeloablative conditioning is typically used for patients with leaky SCID and Omenn's syndrome and those with functional NKs (e.g., RAG1/2, Artemis). Conversely, patients with T−B+ SCID (e.g., IL2RG, JAK3) usually do not require myeloablative chemotherapy, as they have a very low barrier to engraftment [4]. In patients with presumed or confirmed radiation-sensitive SCID, sensitivity to alkylating agents must be kept in mind for choosing the best strategy, and a definitive diagnosis is essential before HSCT [24].

4.3.3 Complications and Late Effects

Infections are the main concern for patients with SCID, before, during, and after HSCT. Infections acquired before transplantation, especially where a newborn screening program is not active, can strongly impact survival both before and soon after HSCT [11, 16]. EBV, CMV, and adenovirus are major concerns, but many other viral agents can be implicated and must be carefully ruled out. Aggressive monitoring strategies (PCR-based) must be put in place to allow prompt interventions. Moreover, post-transplant lymphoproliferative disease can be a serious, though rare, consequence of EBV proliferation after HSCT. Acute and chronic GvHD still represent a significant concern, accounting for around 20% and 15% of cases, respectively [11, 16]. As previously mentioned, GvHD prevention strategies mostly consist of T-cell depletion (in vivo and ex vivo). Direct toxicity of treatments, mostly the myeloablative regimens, can induce severe and life-threatening organ damage, especially at the liver (veno-occlusive disease) and lung levels. Rejection of the graft is another critical issue, especially in some SCID subtypes when there is a residual T-cell or NK function, and usually requires a second HSCT (from the same or a different donor). The choice of the best conditioning regimen according to the diagnosis and the risk of rejection is therefore essential [11]. Immune reconstitution should be monitored through lymphocyte evaluation (naive and memory T-cell, NK-cell, and B-cell subsets). Finally, autoimmune hemolytic anemia (prompted by ABO group incompatibility) and other autoimmunity disorders are other potential complications that require (even prolonged) immunosuppressive treatment.

In addition to late effects that occur in all patients receiving HSCT (e.g., endocrine abnormalities, cognitive deficits, pulmonary dysfunction, malignancies), HSCT carries specific risks in patients with SCID. Among them, infections, growth retard and nutritional deficits, autoimmune or inflammatory manifestations, and chronic HPV infection must be carefully investigated, as well as specific features such as neurocognitive consequences that can also be a direct consequence of the specific SCID defect [25].

4.4 Gene Therapy

Despite allogeneic HSCT being a curative approach for SCID, it bears procedure-related mortality and long-term complications associated with GVHD and myeloablative regimens. To overcome these limitations, in the last two decades, gene therapy has been developed and perfected as a safe alternative to allogeneic HSCT.

Gene therapy exploits the intrinsic ability of retroviruses to integrate into the host genome, using these genetically engineered viruses as vectors to add the correct copy of the disease-causing gene to the patient's own cells. Previous trials utilized viral particles derived from a gamma-retrovirus as a vector. However, these vectors carried strong gene promoters that, when sporadically integrated close to the host proto-oncogene, could increase the likelihood of developing leukemia years after treatment [26]. To overcome this issue, gamma-retroviruses have been replaced by self-inactivating lentiviral vectors, which feature lower genotoxicity and are more easily transduced [27].

In more detail, autologous hematopoietic stem cells (HSCs) expressing the CD34+ surface marker are harvested and transduced ex vivo with the viral vector engineered to be non-self-replicating and to encode the complementary DNA (cDNA) of the therapeutic gene. Within the cells, the RNA of the virus undergoes reverse transcription to DNA and integrates into the host genome. Meanwhile, the patient undergoes a non-myeloablative conditioning regimen to open the bone marrow niches, essentially making space for the new cells to engraft. The transduced HSCs are infused back into the patient, where they begin to proliferate and differentiate, leading to the repopulation of the immune compartment with cells expressing the therapeutic gene.

This approach, based on the use of patient-derived cells, brings several advantages: it is virtually available to every patient and eliminates the risk of developing GVHD. Additionally, the introduction of new antigenic material is minimal, thus lowering the risk of graft rejection. Moreover, it is possible to achieve engraftment with non-myeloablative conditioning regimens, which proves especially useful for SCID sensitive to alkylating agent-mediated DNA damage, such as ARTEMIS SCID [27, 28].

Currently, gene therapy has proven to be a safe and effective alternative for Adenosine Deaminase Deficiency (ADA)-SCID, X-linked SCID, and ARTEMIS SCID in patients without an available HLA-matched donor. Follow-up studies have confirmed long-term survival and immune reconstitution in patients who underwent gene therapy [28–31].

Despite its success, gene therapy is associated with side effects. Even though self-inactivating lentiviral vectors have a better safety profile, the procedure is inherently genotoxic due to the insertional mutagenesis process. As a result, patients may develop leukemia and myelodysplasia even years after receiving the treatment. Another side effect that has been observed is the occurrence of autoimmunity, mainly autoimmune anemia, which tends to occur transiently during the phase of immune reconstitution. It is noteworthy that the use of new lentiviral vectors is relatively recent, and thus, the follow-up period is limited; long-term safety and efficacy data are still being gathered and will need to be compared to the long-term results of HSCT.

One of the significant limitations of gene therapy is its extreme cost and limited access, which is mainly restricted to clinical trials and specialized centers equipped to handle complex ex vivo procedures. The advancements in this technology have opened up an exciting chapter of research aimed at overcoming current limits and extending gene therapy to other conditions, by for example exploring the fields of gene editing and in vivo gene therapy.

4.5 Conclusions

The clinical management of SCID is a complex landscape in continuous evolution. Many goals have been reached in the last decades, mostly by improving transplant strategy and introducing newborn screening. Moreover, gene therapy is now both a solid reality and a promising frontier. However, patients with SCID still face many challenges and morbidities. In the future, further improvements in their prognosis will surely depend on the optimization and extension of the screening programs, on more personalized management strategies based on the patient's genetic and clinical characteristics, and on the extension of gene therapy approaches to more genetic defects.

References

1. Bonilla FA, Khan DA, Ballas ZK, Chinen J, Frank MM, Hsu JT, Keller M, Kobrynski LJ, Komarow HD, Mazer B, Nelson RP Jr, Orange JS, Routes JM, Shearer WT, Sorensen RU, Verbsky JW, Bernstein DI, Blessing-Moore J, Lang D, Nicklas RA, Oppenheimer J, Portnoy JM, Randolph CR, Schuller D, Spector SL, Tilles S, Wallace D, Joint Task Force on Practice Parameters, representing the American Academy of Allergy, Asthma & Immunology; the American College of Allergy, Asthma & Immunology; and the Joint Council of Allergy, Asthma & Immunology (2015) Practice parameter for the diagnosis and management of primary immunodeficiency. J Allergy Clin Immunol 136(5):1186–205.e1–78
2. Lankester AC, Albert MH, Booth C, Gennery AR, Güngör T, Hönig M, Morris EC, Moshous D, Neven B, Schulz A, Slatter M, Veys P, Inborn Errors Working Party of the European Society for Blood and Marrow Transplantation and the European Society for Immune Deficiencies, and European Reference Network on Rare Primary Immunodeficiency Autoinflammatory Autoimmune diseases (RITA) (2021) EBMT/ESID inborn errors working party guidelines for hematopoietic stem cell transplantation for inborn errors of immunity. Bone Marrow Transplant 56(9):2052–2062
3. Slatter MA, Gennery AR (2022) Advances in the treatment of severe combined immunodeficiency. Clin Immunol 242:109084
4. Dorsey MJ, Dvorak CC, Cowan MJ, Puck JM (2017) Treatment of infants identified as having severe combined immunodeficiency by means of newborn screening. J Allergy Clin Immunol 139:733
5. Perez EE, Orange JS, Bonilla F, Chinen J, Chinn IK, Dorsey M, El-Gamal Y, Harville TO, Hossny E, Mazer B, Nelson R, Secord E, Jordan SC, Stiehm ER, Vo AA, Ballow M (2017) Update on the use of immunoglobulin in human disease: a review of evidence. J Allergy Clin Immunol 139(3S):S1–S46
6. American Academy of Pediatrics Committee on Infectious Diseases; American Academy of Pediatrics Bronchiolitis Guidelines Committee (2014) Updated guidance for palivizumab prophylaxis among infants and young children at increased risk of hospitalization for respiratory syncytial virus infection. Pediatrics 134(2):e620–e638
7. Medical Advisory Committee of the Immune Deficiency Foundation, Shearer WT, Fleisher TA, Buckley RH, Ballas Z, Ballow M, Blaese RM, Bonilla FA, Conley ME, Cunningham-Rundles C, Filipovich AH, Fuleihan R, Gelfand EW, Hernandez-Trujillo V, Holland SM, Hong R, Lederman HM, Malech HL, Miles S, Notarangelo LD, Ochs HD, Orange JS, Puck JM, Routes JM, Stiehm ER, Sullivan K, Torgerson T, Winkelstein J (2014) Recommendations for live viral and bacterial vaccines in immunodeficient patients and their close contacts. J Allergy Clin Immunol 133(4):961–966
8. Kimberlin DW (2024) Red Book: 2024 Report of the Committee on Infectious Diseases, 33rd edn. American Academy of Pediatrics
9. Rivers L, Gaspar HB (2015) Severe combined immunodeficiency: recent developments and guidance on clinical management. Arch Dis Child 100(7):667–672
10. Lankester AC, Neven B, Mahlaoui N, von Asmuth EGJ, Courteille V, Alligon M, Albert MH, Serra IB, Bader P, Balashov D, Beier R, Bertrand Y, Blanche S, Bordon V, Bredius RG, Cant A, Cavazzana M, Diaz-de-Heredia C, Dogu F, Ehlert K, Entz-Werle N, Fasth A, Ferrua F,

Ferster A, Formankova R, Friedrich W, Gonzalez-Vicent M, Gozdzik J, Güngör T, Hoenig M, Ikinciogullari A, Kalwak K, Kansoy S, Kupesiz A, Lanfranchi A, Lindemans CA, Meisel R, Michel G, Miranda NAA, Moraleda J, Moshous D, Pichler H, Rao K, Sedlacek P, Slatter M, Soncini E, Speckmann C, Sundin M, Toren A, Vettenranta K, Worth A, Yeşilipek MA, Zecca M, Porta F, Schulz A, Veys P, Fischer A, Gennery AR (2022) Hematopoietic cell transplantation in severe combined immunodeficiency: the SCETIDE 2006–2014 European cohort. J Allergy Clin Immunol 149(5):1744–1754.e8

11. Pai SY, Logan BR, Griffith LM, Buckley RH, Parrott RE, Dvorak CC, Kapoor N, Hanson IC, Filipovich AH, Jyonouchi S, Sullivan KE, Small TN, Burroughs L, Skoda-Smith S, Haight AE, Grizzle A, Pulsipher MA, Chan KW, Fuleihan RL, Haddad E, Loechelt B, Aquino VM, Gillio A, Davis J, Knutsen A, Smith AR, Moore TB, Schroeder ML, Goldman FD, Connelly JA, Porteus MH, Xiang Q, Shearer WT, Fleisher TA, Kohn DB, Puck JM, Notarangelo LD, Cowan MJ, O'Reilly RJ (2014) Transplantation outcomes for severe combined immunodeficiency, 2000–2009. N Engl J Med 371(5):434–446
12. Myers LA, Patel DD, Puck JM, Buckley RH (2002) Hematopoietic stem cell transplantation for severe combined immunodeficiency in the neonatal period leads to superior thymic output and improved survival. Blood 99(3):872–878
13. Railey MD, Lokhnygina Y, Buckley RH (2009) Long-term clinical outcome of patients with severe combined immunodeficiency who received related donor bone marrow transplants without pretransplant chemotherapy or post-transplant GVHD prophylaxis. J Pediatr 155(6):834–840.e1
14. Thakar MS, Logan BR, Puck JM, Dunn EA, Buckley RH, Cowan MJ, O'Reilly RJ, Kapoor N, Satter LF, Pai SY, Heimall J, Chandra S, Ebens CL, Chellapandian D, Williams O, Burroughs LM, Saldana BD, Rayes A, Madden LM, Chandrakasan S, Bednarski JJ II, DeSantes KB, Cuvelier GDE, Teira P, Gillio AP, Eissa H, Knutsen AP, Goldman FD, Aquino VM, Shereck EB, Moore TB, Caywood EH, Lugt MTV, Rozmus J, Broglie L, Yu LC, Shah AJ, Andolina JR, Liu X, Parrott RE, Dara J, Prockop S, Martinez CA, Kapadia M, Jyonouchi SC, Sullivan KE, Bleesing JJ, Chaudhury S, Petrovic A, Keller MD, Quigg TC, Parikh S, Shenoy S, Seroogy C, Rubin T, Decaluwe H, Routes JM, Torgerson TR, Leiding JW, Pulsipher MA, Kohn DB, Griffith LM, Haddad E, Dvorak CC, Notarangelo LD (2023) Measuring the effect of newborn screening on survival after haematopoietic cell transplantation for severe combined immunodeficiency: a 36-year longitudinal study from the Primary Immune Deficiency Treatment Consortium. Lancet 402(10396):129–140
15. Gaspar HB, Aiuti A, Porta F et al (2009) How I treat ADA deficiency. Blood 114:3524
16. Heimall J, Logan BR, Cowan MJ, Notarangelo LD, Griffith LM, Puck JM, Kohn DB, Pulsipher MA, Parikh S, Martinez C, Kapoor N, O'Reilly R, Boyer M, Pai SY, Goldman F, Burroughs L, Chandra S, Kletzel M, Thakar M, Connelly J, Cuvelier G, Davila Saldana BJ, Shereck E, Knutsen A, Sullivan KE, DeSantes K, Gillio A, Haddad E, Petrovic A, Quigg T, Smith AR, Stenger E, Yin Z, Shearer WT, Fleisher T, Buckley RH, Dvorak CC (2017) Immune reconstitution and survival of 100 SCID patients post-hematopoietic cell transplant: a PIDTC natural history study. Blood 130(25):2718–2727
17. Grunebaum E, Mazzolari E, Porta F, Dallera D, Atkinson A, Reid B, Notarangelo LD, Roifman CM (2006) Bone marrow transplantation for severe combined immune deficiency. JAMA 295(5):508–518
18. Dvorak CC, Hassan A, Slatter MA, Hönig M, Lankester AC, Buckley RH, Pulsipher MA, Davis JH, Güngör T, Gabriel M, Bleesing JH, Bunin N, Sedlacek P, Connelly JA, Crawford DF, Notarangelo LD, Pai SY, Hassid J, Veys P, Gennery AR, Cowan MJ (2014) Comparison of outcomes of hematopoietic stem cell transplantation without chemotherapy conditioning by using matched sibling and unrelated donors for treatment of severe combined immunodeficiency. J Allergy Clin Immunol 134(4):935–943.e15
19. Ramanathan S, Lum SH, Nademi Z, Carruthers K, Watson H, Flood T, Owens S, Williams E, Hambleton S, Gennery AR, Slatter M (2023) CD3+TCRαβ/CD19+-depleted mismatched family or unrelated donor salvage stem cell transplantation for graft dysfunction in inborn errors of immunity. Transplant Cell Ther 29(8):513.e1–513.e9
20. Fernandes JF, Rocha V, Labopin M, Neven B, Moshous D, Gennery AR, Friedrich W, Porta F, Diaz de Heredia C, Wall D, Bertrand Y, Veys P, Slatter M, Schulz A, Chan KW, Grimley M,

Ayas M, Gungor T, Ebell W, Bonfim C, Kalwak K, Taupin P, Blanche S, Gaspar HB, Landais P, Fischer A, Gluckman E, Cavazzana-Calvo M; Eurocord and Inborn Errors Working Party of European Group for Blood and Marrow Transplantation. Transplantation in patients with SCID: mismatched related stem cells or unrelated cord blood? Blood. 2012;119(12):2949–2955

21. Admiraal R, Lindemans CA, van Kesteren C, Bierings MB, Versluijs AB, Nierkens S, Boelens JJ (2016) Excellent T-cell reconstitution and survival depend on low ATG exposure after pediatric cord blood transplantation. Blood 128(23):2734–2741
22. Rao K, Amrolia PJ, Jones A, Cale CM, Naik P, King D, Davies GE, Gaspar HB, Veys PA (2005) Improved survival after unrelated donor bone marrow transplantation in children with primary immunodeficiency using a reduced-intensity conditioning regimen. Blood 105(2):879–885
23. Slatter MA, Rao K, Abd Hamid IJ, Nademi Z, Chiesa R, Elfeky R, Pearce MS, Amrolia P, Worth A, Flood T, Abinun M, Hambleton S, Qasim W, Gaspar HB, Cant AJ, Gennery AR, Veys P (2018) Treosulfan and fludarabine conditioning for hematopoietic stem cell transplantation in children with primary immunodeficiency: UK experience. Biol Blood Marrow Transplant 24(3):529–536
24. Cowan MJ, Gennery AR (2015) Radiation-sensitive severe combined immunodeficiency: the arguments for and against conditioning before hematopoietic cell transplantation—what to do? J Allergy Clin Immunol 136(5):1178–1185
25. Neven B, Leroy S, Decaluwe H, Le Deist F, Picard C, Moshous D, Mahlaoui N, Debré M, Casanova JL, Dal Cortivo L, Madec Y, Hacein-Bey-Abina S, de Saint Basile G, de Villartay JP, Blanche S, Cavazzana-Calvo M, Fischer A (2009) Long-term outcome after hematopoietic stem cell transplantation of a single-center cohort of 90 patients with severe combined immunodeficiency. Blood 113(17):4114–4124
26. Hacein-Bey-Abina S, Garrigue A, Wang GP, Soulier J, Lim A, Morillon E, Clappier E, Caccavelli L, Delabesse E, Beldjord K, Asnafi V, MacIntyre E, Dal Cortivo L, Radford I, Brousse N, Sigaux F, Moshous D, Hauer J, Borkhardt A, Belohradsky BH, Wintergerst U, Velez MC, Leiva L, Sorensen R, Wulffraat N, Blanche S, Bushman FD, Fischer A, Cavazzana-Calvo M (2008) Insertional oncogenesis in 4 patients after retrovirus-mediated gene therapy of SCID-X1. J Clin Invest 118(9):3132–3142. https://doi.org/10.1172/JCI35700
27. Naldini L, Cicalese MP, Bernardo ME, Gentner B, Gabaldo M, Ferrari G, Aiuti A (2022) The EHA research roadmap: hematopoietic stem cell gene therapy. Hemasphere 6(2):e671. https://doi.org/10.1097/HS9.0000000000000671
28. Cowan MJ, Yu J, Facchino J, Fraser-Browne C, Sanford U, Kawahara M, Dara J, Long-Boyle J, Oh J, Chan W, Chag S, Broderick L, Chellapandian D, Decaluwe H, Golski C, Hu D, Kuo CY, Miller HK, Petrovic A, Currier R, Hilton JF, Punwani D, Dvorak CC, Malech HL, McIvor RS, Puck JM (2022) Lentiviral gene therapy for Artemis-deficient SCID. N Engl J Med 387(25):2344–2355. https://doi.org/10.1056/NEJMoa2206575
29. Reinhardt B, Habib O, Shaw KL, Garabedian E, Carbonaro-Sarracino DA, Terrazas D, Fernandez BC, De Oliveira S, Moore TB, Ikeda AK, Engel BC, Podsakoff GM, Hollis RP, Fernandes A, Jackson C, Shupien S, Mishra S, Davila A, Mottahedeh J, Vitomirov A, Meng W, Rosenfeld AM, Roche AM, Hokama P, Reddy S, Everett J, Wang X, Luning Prak ET, Cornetta K, Hershfield MS, Sokolic R, De Ravin SS, Malech HL, Bushman FD, Candotti F, Kohn DB (2021) Long-term outcomes after gene therapy for adenosine deaminase severe combined immune deficiency. Blood 138(15):1304–1316. https://doi.org/10.1182/blood.2020010260
30. Hacein-Bey-Abina S, Hauer J, Lim A, Picard C, Wang GP, Berry CC, Martinache C, Rieux-Laucat F, Latour S, Belohradsky BH, Leiva L, Sorensen R, Debré M, Casanova JL, Blanche S, Durandy A, Bushman FD, Fischer A, Cavazzana-Calvo M (2010) Efficacy of gene therapy for X-linked severe combined immunodeficiency. N Engl J Med 363(4):355–364. https://doi.org/10.1056/NEJMoa1000164
31. Mamcarz E, Zhou S, Lockey T, Abdelsamed H, Cross SJ, Kang G, Ma Z, Condori J, Dowdy J, Triplett B, Li C, Maron G, Aldave Becerra JC, Church JA, Dokmeci E, Love JT, da Matta Ain AC, van der Watt H, Tang X, Janssen W, Ryu BY, De Ravin SS, Weiss MJ, Youngblood B, Long-Boyle JR, Gottschalk S, Meagher MM, Malech HL, Puck JM, Cowan MJ, Sorrentino BP (2019) Lentiviral gene therapy combined with low-dose busulfan in infants with SCID-X1. N Engl J Med 380(16):1525–1534. https://doi.org/10.1056/NEJMoa1815408

Hot Topics in Severe Combined Immunodeficiency (SCID)

5

Sofia D'Elios, Mario Milco D'Elios, and Nagaja Capitani

5.1 Introduction

Severe combined immunodeficiency (SCID) is the most severe primary immune deficiency, consisting of a heterogeneous group of genetic defects affecting the immune system development and function. The overall frequency is estimated to 1 in 40,000 to 75,000 newborns and despite it is a prenatal disorder, frequently SCID is observed in the first few months of life and the median age at diagnosis is 4–7 months [1].

SCID is mainly characterized by impaired differentiation of both $CD4^+$ and $CD8^+$ T lymphocytes, that is variably associated with defects in other lymphocyte lineages, such as B lymphocytes or natural killer (NK) cells, or more rarely in the myeloid lineage [2, 3]. Based on the immunological defects, SCID can be classified into the following subgroups depending on the presence of further B or NK defects: $T^- B^+ NK^+$, $T^- B^+ NK^-$, $T^- B^- NK^+$, $T^- B^- NK^-$. This immunophenotypic classification is usually associated with specific gene defects (genotypes), which are in turn associated with a variety of clinical manifestation.

Here we summarized the main SCID subsets, recapitulating the principal genes affected and the associated clinical course, and we give an overview of the classical therapeutic approaches, together with the new frontiers in SCID treatment.

S. D'Elios
Department of Clinical and Experimental Medicine, University of Pisa, Pisa, Italy

M. M. D'Elios (✉)
Department of Molecular and Developmental Medicine, University of Siena, Siena, Italy
e-mail: delios@unisi.it

N. Capitani (✉)
Department of Life Sciences, University of Siena, Siena, Italy
e-mail: capitani2@unisi.it

M. M. D'Elios (ed.), *Severe Combined Immunodeficiency*, Rare Diseases of the Immune System, https://doi.org/10.1007/978-3-031-78864-2_5

5.2 Genotype/Phenotype and Clinical Aspects of SCID

5.2.1 $T^- B^+ NK^+$ Subset

In approximately 10% of SCID patients characterized by compromised T-cell development with normal B and NK functions, mutations impairing the expression of the α subunit of the IL-7 receptor have been described (*IL-7Rα*) [4]. IL-7R is a heterodimeric receptor and consists of two subunits, IL-7Rα (CD127) and common gamma chain (γc) receptor. Signaling mediated by the cytokine interleukin 7 (IL-7) following the binding with IL-7R is essential for the differentiation of T cells from the lymphoid progenitors. In SCID patients, a number of mutation sites for *IL-7R* gene have been identified, including three nucleotide substitutions that resulted in missense mutations, one nonsense mutation, and one substitution associate with a splicing site mutation [4]. In this type of SCID, the defective gene prevents the creation of the IL-7R receptor chain, which interrupts the downstream signaling pathways, with severe effects on T cells development (Fig. 5.1). Patients with IL-7R defects present in early infancy a classic SCID phenotype: failure to thrive (FTT), diarrhea, severe thrush, *Pneumocystis jiroveci* pneumonia, and severe viral respiratory infections.

5.2.2 $T^- B^+ NK^-$ Subset

5.2.2.1 Common Gamma Chain (γc) Defect

X-linked severe combined immunodeficiency (X-SCID) is an immunodeficiency disorder that accounts for about half of the cases of SCID, and it is characterized by an absence of mature T and NK cells, whereas B cells have a normal phenotype [5]. It is an X-linked recessive inheritance trait caused by mutations of *IL2RG* gene, localized at Xq13.1 and encoding the γc of interleukin 2 (IL-2) receptor (IL-2R). IL-2R γc is shared by other interleukin receptors such as the receptor for IL-4, IL-7, IL-9, IL-15, and IL-21 [6]; in particular, IL-7- and IL-15-derived pathways are essential for the development of T lymphocytes and NK cells, respectively [7]. Mutation in *IL2RG* gene observed in SCID patients were first described in 1993 [8, 9], and since then, there have been identified more than 200 mutations in the 8 exons of the gene, mainly frameshift mutations [10] (Fig. 5.1).

Infants before 3 months of age affected by X-SCID often show infections due to the decreased amount of immunoglobulin G (IgG) levels [11], followed by viral infections such as pneumonitis, with common symptoms such as cough, fever, chills, and shortness of breath [12], or fungal infection caused, for example, by *Candida albicans* [13]. Other common infections experienced by individuals with X-SCID include diarrhea, sepsis, and otitis media [11].

5.2.2.2 JAK3 (Janus Kinase 3) Deficiency

A non-X-linked form of SCID characterized by a phenotype identical to X-SCID has been shown to be associated with *JAK3* encoding gene mutations [14, 15].

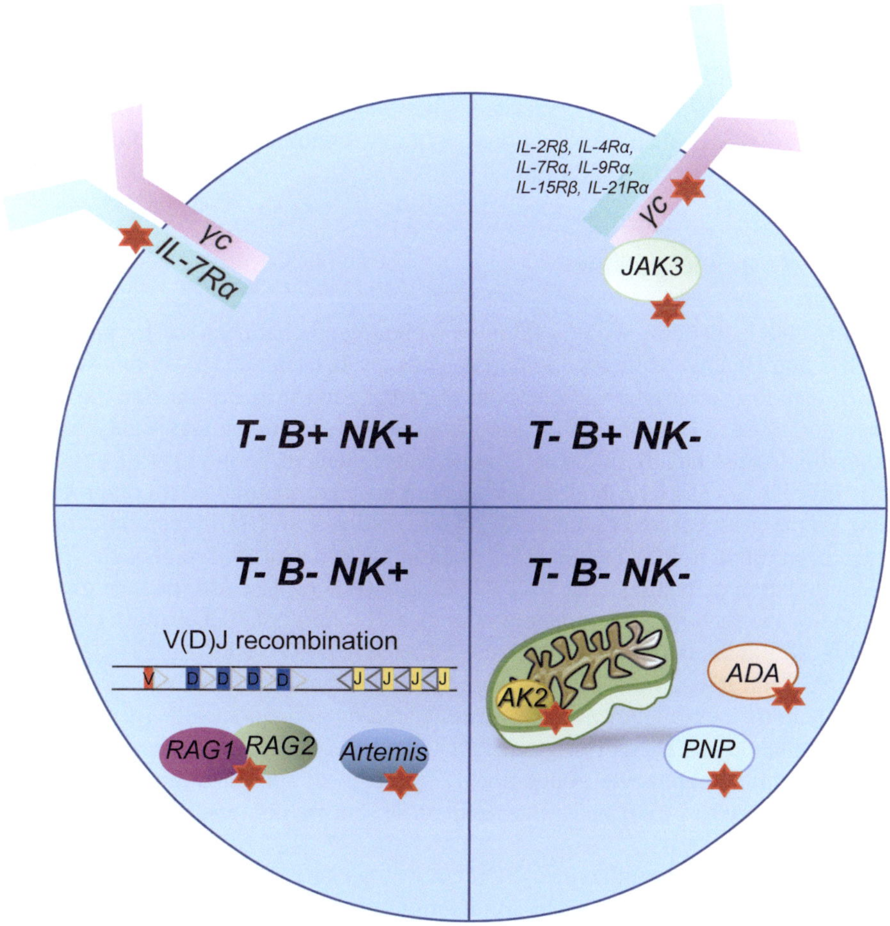

Fig. 5.1 Immunophenotypes in SCID. SCID results from a diverse group of mutations impacting T-cell development, and it is diagnosed and classified through assessment of the lymphocyte subset(s) affected

Janus kinase 3 (JAK3) is a tyrosine kinase that belongs to the Janus family of kinases. JAK3 binds to the intracellular tail of γc subunit and is activated upon cytokine binding to the receptor. Once activated, JAK3 recruits and phosphorylates STAT-5 transcription factor that dimerize, translocate to the nucleus, bind DNA and induce expression of specific genes involved in T and NK cell development [16]. JAK3-deficient SCID accounts for an estimated 7–14% of SCID cases.

Because of the key role of JAK3 in the signaling pathway downstream the common γc subunit and due to the multiple cytokines using this pathway, an early and severe block in T and NK cell development is typically observed in SCID patients with JAK3 deficiency.

A number of distinct mutations in *JAK3* gene were observed in SCID patients, most leading to premature stop codon, with the production of a nonfunctional protein [17] (Fig. 5.1). Affected infants typically develop chronic diarrhea, oral thrush, pneumonia, and skin rashes. Persistent illness also causes affected individuals to grow more slowly than other children. Without treatment, JAK3-deficient SCID patients usually live for a short time.

5.2.3 $T^- B^- NK^+$ Subset

About 20% of patients with SCID have a phenotype characterized by a defect in both T and B cells, while functional NK cells are detectable [18]. In this subset of SCID patients, a number of defects have been found in genes involved in V(D)J recombination, a key process for the generation of functional and highly variable immunoglobulin and T-cell receptor gene rearrangement. In the light of this, when this process is defective, both B and T lymphocytes maturation is compromised. Two of the most common mutations in gene involved in V(D)J recombination that have been found in SCID patients are mutation in genes of the lymphocyte-specific recombination activating gene 1 (RAG1) and 2 (RAG2) [19, 20], and the mutation in one of the factors of the nonhomologous end joining (NHEJ) pathway of DNA double-strand break repair, the nuclease DCLRE1C/ARTEMIS [21, 22].

RAG1 and RAG2 initiate the process of V(D)J recombination and play an essential role in the rearrangement of the genes encoding antigen-specific receptors of B and T lymphocytes, thereby originating a wide variety of receptor repertoire present in the mature lymphocyte population [23]. Many of the mutations in RAG1 or RAG2 observed in SCID patients result in absent or nonfunctional protein [24] (Fig. 5.1).

Clinically, patients with typical SCID show high susceptibility to life-threatening viral, fungal, parasitic, and bacterial infections since early after birth [25]. To note that patients with hypomorphic mutations in RAG1 or RAG2 that maintain partial V(D)J recombination activity can give rise to a wide spectrum of clinical and immunological phenotypes, ranging from Omenn syndrome (OS) to atypical SCID [26, 27].

Artemis defect, indeed, is due to mutations of the *DCLRE1C* (DNA cross-link repair protein 1C) gene, that encodes for Artemis protein. This is a structure-specific DNA endonuclease responsible for hairpin opening in V(D)J recombination and it contributes to end-processing in NHEJ DNA repair. A large number of mutations in *DCLRE1C* were observed in all world populations, with the most common of these known as "SCIDA," that is SCID of Athabaskan-speaking Native Americans (Apache, Navajo), mainly accounting for Artemis loss-of-function [28] (Fig. 5.1).

Artemis mutations cause problems similar to other syndromes with DNA repair defects, such as recurrent respiratory tract infections, candidiasis, immune dysregulation, predisposition to neoplasia, and, in some case, dysmorphic facies, microcephaly, and psychomotor delay. Patients with hypomorphic mutations in *DCLRE1C* gene display less severe clinical courses, such as a mere antibody deficiency [29].

5.2.4 T⁻ B⁻ NK⁻ Subset

This subset of SCID patient represents the cases where not only B and T cell development is affected, but also NK maturation and function are compromised. Are part of this category patients with reticular dysgenesis (RD) and patients with deficiency in adenosine deaminase (ADA-SCID) or purine nucleoside phosphorylase (PNP-SCID).

5.2.4.1 Reticular Dysgenesis (RD)

RD is caused by mutations in the *AK2* gene, located on chromosome 1p35.1, encoding the mitochondrial enzyme adenylate kinase 2 (AK2) [30]. AK2 is a phosphotransferase enzyme localized in the mitochondrial intermembrane space and catalyzes the reversible transfer of a phosphoryl group from adenosine triphosphate (ATP) to adenosine monophosphate (AMP), giving two adenosine diphosphate (ADP) molecules [31]. This is a critical process for cellular energy and homeostasis, and it has a key role in differentiation and proliferation of hematopoietic stem cells. Mutations observed in *AK2* gene from SCID patients include missense mutations or deletion that generates a premature stop codon [32] (Fig. 5.1).

Reticular dysgenesis accounts for less than 2% of all SCID cases, and it represents the most severe form of SCID, characterized by bilateral sensorineural deafness and a lack of innate and adaptive immune functions leading to fatal septicemia within days after birth if not treated [32].

5.2.4.2 Adenosine Deaminase Deficiency (ADA-SCID) and Purine Nucleoside Phosphorylase Deficiency (PNP-SCID)

Deficiency of adenosine deaminase is a cause of human SCID, and it is associated with mutations in *ADA* gene. Adenosine deaminase is a key enzyme of the purine metabolism pathway which catalyzes the irreversible deamination of adenosine and deoxyadenosine to inosine and deoxyinosine, respectively [33]. In mammalian cells, ADA regulates a series of reactions, with a key role in the differentiation and maturation of the lymphoid system [34]. About 20% of SCIDs are caused by ADA deficiency, with an estimated incidence of 1 in 500,000 [35]. A large variety of mutations occurring in the *ADA* gene have been found in SCID patients, resulting in single amino acid substitutions, premature stop codons, RNA splicing errors, insertions and deletions or defects in post-translational modification of the protein [36]. The disease is caused by the intracellular accumulation of adenosine and dAdo substrates that are indirectly toxic to lymphocytes [37, 38] (Fig. 5.1).

Clinical manifestations in ADA-SCID often occur earlier than in other forms of SCID, even if in some cases a late onset was observed, depending on the genetic defect. Together with severe infections and FTT, approximately 50% of ADA-SCID patients develop also skeletal abnormalities and neurological signs [39].

Similarly to what observed for ADA deficiency, another enzyme known as purine nucleoside phosphorylase (PNP) plays a key role in SCID. PNP is a key enzyme in the purine pathway, required for purine degradation. Specifically, it catalyzes the degradation of the nucleosides, inosine, and guanosine, or their deoxy-analog to the corresponding bases. A PNP deficiency leads to elevated deoxy-GTP (dGTP) levels resulting in T-cell toxicity and deficiency.

PNP deficiency in SCID is caused by mutations in the *PNP* gene, resulting in the reduction or abrogation of its enzymatic activity. Among the most common mutations observed in SCID patients, there are point mutations leading to amino acid substitutions [40–42], and splicing defects leading to an inactive, truncated gene product [43] (Fig. 5.1). Clinically, PNP-SCID is characterized by immunological defects as observed for the majority of SCID cases, often associated with neurological problems including developmental delay, hypertonia, spasticity, tremors, ataxia, retarded motor development [44].

5.3 SCID Diagnosis and Therapeutic Principles

Early diagnosis of SCID is extremely important because treating the disease in the first months of life offers a higher probability of survival for children. Until a few years ago, indeed, many SCID children were not diagnosed until sixth months of life, and they died in early childhood after repeated infections. Today, thanks to advanced diagnosis methods, such as prenatal diagnosis or newborn screening, children with SCID can be successfully treated.

Among the prenatal diagnosis methods there are the identification of mutation in genes involved in SCID by chorionic villous biopsy at week 8–10 of gestation or in other cases, the analyses of fetal lymphocyte populations in the cord blood taken under echography at week 20–22 of gestation. Together with these prenatal diagnosis methods, newborn screening panels for SCID are available and they are of particularly relevance to determine the type of SCID and to guide treatment recommendations [45].

Usually hematopoietic stem cell transplantation (HSCT) or gene therapy represent the elective treatments for SCID. In the absence of such therapy, patients usually die, except for ADA-deficient SCID patients for which enzyme replacement by PEG-ADA may result in prolonged survival [38] (Fig. 5.2).

5.3.1 Hematopoietic Stem Cell Transplantation (HSCT)

HSCT is the most efficient treatment option for SCID infants. The objective of HSCT in SCID patients is to provide healthy hematopoietic stem cells, allowing immune defect correction. Stem cells are usually obtained from the bone marrow or other blood components of a healthy donor and once transplanted, they originate healthy T and B cells inside the host, restoring a functional immunological repertoire. Transplantations carried out within first 3 months after birth have been reported to be the most successful [46–49], with an overall survival of 85–90% [50, 51].

However, the outcome of HSCT for SCID is related to a number of different factors. The factor with most impact on survival was the donor category, more in detail it is related to the type and degree of human leukocyte antigen (HLA) match of the

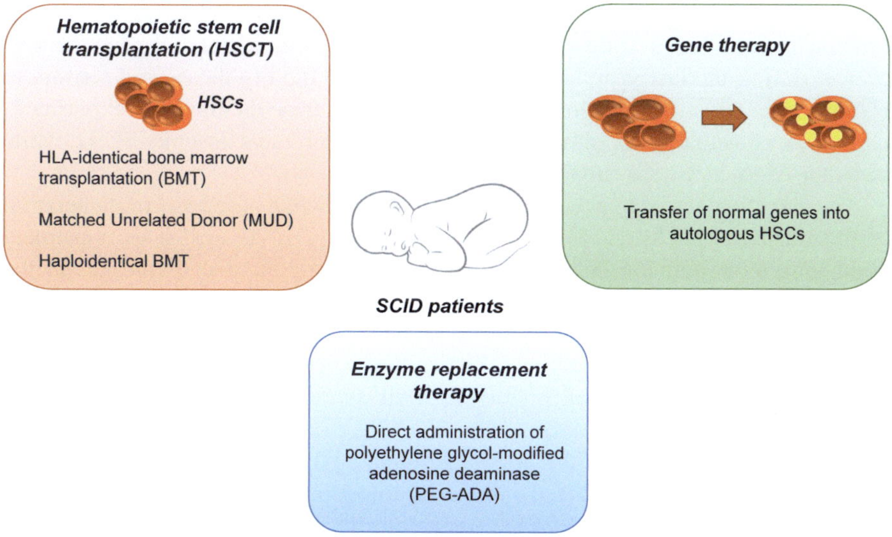

Fig. 5.2 Current therapeutic options in SCID. Immune reconstitution in SCID patients can be achieved by bone marrow transplantation, gene therapy or, for a subset of patient, by enzyme replacement

donor. The most promising and successful donor type is certainly represented by the matched sibling donor (MSD), followed by haploidentical donor and matched unrelated donor (MUD) [49, 52]. Unfortunately, MSD are found for only 15–25% of patients, which is why the need to look for other donor sources and in particular the use of haploidentical donor that in the recent years is becoming one of the most promising alternatives [53].

The outcome of HSCT for SCID is furthermore related to other different factors, among which an important role is played by the SCID genotype and the conditioning regimen. To note, survival in patients with RAG mutations was significantly better than in patients with DCLRE1C mutations, despite being both T^- B^- NK^+ phenotypes [54]. At the same time, the role of conditioning regimen (chemotherapy, monoclonal antibody therapy, and radiation) in HSCT for SCID remains controversial, with absence of chemotherapy-induced toxicity to one end and successful engraftment to the other end [55, 56].

5.3.2 Gene Therapy

The characterization of a panel of SCID-associated genes opens the field to another less common but promising new treatment option, the gene therapy. It is basically an autologous HSCT accompanied to gene editing: defective stem cells are isolated from an SCID patient, manipulated *ex vivo* for the introduction of the healthy copy of the human gene of interest and then transplanted back into the patient. This "corrected" version of cells further divide and proliferate, restoring a working immune system. Retroviruses are usually employed as the vectors for gene therapy, even if during the last years attempts were made to modify these viral vectors to obtain a safer but still efficacious process. Nowadays, gene therapy is an experimental treatment available for children with X-linked SCID and Artemis SCID, while trials for ADA-SCID are currently on hold.

The first clinical trial of gene therapy for X-linked SCID, based on first-generation gammaretroviral vectors, was performed in the early 2000s and it demonstrated good long-term immune reconstitution, especially for the T-cell lineage, in the majority of patients, despite few cases of vector-related leukemia [57]. More recently, other clinical trials for X-linked SCID were done or are still ongoing with the perspective to develop new generation and safer vectors such as self-inactivating gammaretroviral or lentiviral vectors as well as major advances in integrome knowledge.

At the same manner, gene therapy for Artemis SCID was developed in the recent years, with a panel of clinical trial based on autologous gene therapy, with the transfer of a normal copy of the *DCLRE1C* gene into stem cells of affected patients.

To note, an advantage of gene therapy compared to HSCT is that it does not warrant a compatible donor and without possibility of host versus graft reactions.

5.3.3 Enzyme Replacement Therapy (ERT)

A third type of treatment can be used in a specific subtype of SCID, the ADA-SCID patients, known as enzyme replacement therapy (ERT). In this type of therapy, the missing ADA enzyme is injected into the SCID patients, resulting in a temporary immune system repair. More in detail, bovine adenosine deaminase is conjugated with polyethylene glycol (PEG) to extend the circulation of ADA enzyme in the blood by increasing the biological half-life of the enzyme [58]. Several studies indicated that intramuscular injection of PEG-ADA biweekly allows an initial differentiation of T lymphocytes from immature thymic precursors and reconstitution of lymphocyte functions [59]. In contrast with this well-documented initial improvement of immunity upon beginning PEG-ADA therapy has been documented, the long-term effects have not been well characterized [60]. In fact, several patients have experienced deterioration in lymphocyte counts and function over time, with higher risk to develop infection and tumors. For these reasons, ERT is often considered a temporary treatment while prompting for HSCT or gene therapy.

5.4 Conclusions and Perspectives

SCID is a severe primary immunodeficiency mainly characterized by impaired differentiation of both $CD4^+$ and $CD8^+$ T lymphocytes and is variably associated with defects in other lymphocyte lineages, such as B lymphocytes or NK cells, or more rarely of the myeloid lineage. Based on the immunological defects, SCID can be classified in the following subgroups depending on the presence of B or NK defects: $T^- B^+ NK^+$, $T^- B^+ NK^-$, $T^- B^- NK^+$, $T^- B^- NK^-$. This immunophenotypic classification is usually associated with specific gene defects (genotypes), which are in turn associated with a variety of clinical manifestation. SCID represents a severe disease that however helped to understand how the immune system functions and which are the main genes and the main functions needed for a healthy immunity. Novel cellular and biological frontiers will be very useful for optimal SCID treatment.

Acknowledgments We thank the University of Siena and the University of Pisa for supporting our studies.

References

1. Chinn IK, Shearer WT (2015) Severe combined immunodeficiency disorders. Immunol Allergy Clin N Am 35:671–694. https://doi.org/10.1016/j.iac.2015.07.002
2. Fischer A, Cavazzana-Calvo M, De Saint Basile G, DeVillartay JP, DiSanto JP, Hivroz C et al (1997) Naturally occurring primary deficiencies of the immune system. Ann Rev Immunol 15:93–124. https://doi.org/10.1146/annurev.immunol.15.1.93
3. Primary immunodeficiency diseases. Report of an IUIS Scientific Committee. International Union of Immunological Societies (1999) Clin Exp Immunol 118(Suppl 1):1–28. https://doi.org/10.1046/j.1365-2249.1999.00109.x
4. Puel A, Ziegler SF, Buckley RH, Leonard WJ (1998) Defective IL7R expression in T(−) B(+) NK(+) severe combined immunodeficiency. Nat Genet 20:394–397. https://doi.org/10.1038/3877
5. Church AC (2002) X-linked severe combined immunodeficiency. Hosp Med 63:676–680. https://doi.org/10.12968/hosp.2002.63.11.1914
6. Puck JM (1996) IL2RGbase: a database of γc-chain defects causing human X-SCID. Immunol Today 17:507–511. https://doi.org/10.1016/0167-5699(96)30062-5
7. Rochman Y, Spolski R, Leonard WJ (2009) New insights into the regulation of T cells by γc family cytokines. Nat Rev Immunol 9:480–490. https://doi.org/10.1038/nri2580
8. Noguchi M, Yi H, Rosenblatt HM, Filipovich AH, Adelstein S, Modi WS et al (1993) Interleukin-2 receptor gamma chain mutation results in X-linked severe combined immunodeficiency in humans. Cell 73:147–157. https://doi.org/10.1016/0092-8674(93)90167-o
9. Puck JM, Deschênes SM, Porter JC, Dutra AS, Brown CJ, Willard HF et al (1993) The interleukin-2 receptor gamma chain maps to Xq13.1 and is mutated in X-linked severe combined immunodeficiency, SCIDX1. Hum Mol Genet 2:1099–1104. https://doi.org/10.1093/hmg/2.8.1099
10. DiSanto JP, Dautry-Varsat A, Certain S, Fischer A, de Saint BG (1994) Interleukin-2 (IL-2) receptor gamma chain mutations in X-linked severe combined immunodeficiency disease result in the loss of high-affinity IL-2 receptor binding. Eur J Immunol 24:475–479. https://doi.org/10.1002/eji.1830240232
11. Vickers P (2009) Severe combined immune deficiency: early hospitalisation and isolation. Wiley, pp 29–47. ISBN 978-0-470-31986-4
12. Sponzilli I, Notarangelo LD (2011) Severe combined immunodeficiency (SCID): from molecular basis to clinical management. Acta Biomed 82:5–13
13. Gennery AR, Cant AJ (2001) Diagnosis of severe combined immunodeficiency. J Clin Pathol 54:191–195. https://doi.org/10.1136/jcp.54.3.191
14. Macchi P, Villa A, Giliani S, Sacco MG, Frattini A, Porta F et al (1995) Mutations of JAK-3 gene in patients with autosomal SCID. Nature 377:65–68. https://doi.org/10.1038/377065a0

15. Russel SM, Tayebi N, Nakajima H, Riedy MC, Roberts JL, Aman MJ et al (1995) Mutation of Jak3 in a patient with SCID: essential role of Jak3 in lymphoid development. Science 270:797–800. https://doi.org/10.1126/science.270.5237.797
16. Ghoreschi K, Laurence A, O'Shea JJ (2009) Janus kinases in immune cell signaling. Immunol Rev 228:273–287. https://doi.org/10.1111/j.1600-065X.2008.00754.x
17. Notarangelo LD, Mella P, Jones A, de Saint Basile G, Savoldi G, Cranston T et al (2001) Mutations in severe combined immune deficiency (SCID) due to JAK3 deficiency. Hum Mutat 18:255–263. https://doi.org/10.1002/humu.1188
18. Buckley RH, Schiff RI, Schiff SE, Markert L, Williams LW, Harvilleto D et al (1997) Human severe combined immunodeficiency: genetic, phenotypic and functional diversity in 100 infants. J Pediatr 130:378–387. https://doi.org/10.1016/s0022-3476(97)70199-9
19. Schwarz K, Gauss GH, Ludwig L, Pannicke U, Li Z, Lindner D et al (1996) RAG mutations in human B cell-negative SCID. Science 274:97–99. https://doi.org/10.1126/science.274.5284.97
20. Sobacchi C, Marrella V, Rucci F, Vezzoni P, Villa A (2006) RAG-dependent primary immunodeficiencies. Hum Mutat 27:1174–1184. https://doi.org/10.1002/humu.20408
21. Moshous D, Callebaut I, de Chasseval R, Corneo B, Cavazzana-Calvo M, Le Deist F et al (2001) Artemis, a novel DNA double-strand break repair/V(D)J recombination protein, is mutated in human severe combined immune deficiency. Cell 105:177–186. https://doi.org/10.1016/s0092-8674(01)00309-9
22. Pannicke U, Hönig M, Schulze I, Rohr J, Heinz GA, Braun S et al (2010) The most frequent DCLRE1C (ARTEMIS) mutations are based on homologous recombination events. Hum Mutat 31:197–207. https://doi.org/10.1002/humu.21168
23. Bassing CH, Swat W, Alt FW (2002) The mechanism and regulation of chromosomal V(D)J recombination. Cell 109(Suppl):S45–S55. https://doi.org/10.1016/s0092-8674(02)00675-x
24. Villa A, Sobacchi C, Notarangelo LD, Bozzi F, Abinun M, Abrahamsen TG et al (2001) V(D)J recombination defects in lymphocytes due to RAG mutations: severe immunodeficiency with a spectrum of clinical presentations. Blood 97:81–88. https://doi.org/10.1182/blood.v97.1.81
25. Delmonte OM, Schuetz C, Notarangelo LD (2018) RAG deficiency: two genes, many diseases. J Clin Immunol 38:646–655. https://doi.org/10.1007/s10875-018-0537-4
26. Villa A, Santagata S, Bozzi F, Imberti L, Notarangelo LD (1999) Omenn syndrome: a disorder of Rag1 and Rag2 genes. J Clin Immunol 19:87–97. https://doi.org/10.1023/a:20550432126
27. Giblin W, Chatterji M, Westfield G, Masud T, Theisen B, Cheng H et al (2009) Leaky severe combined immunodeficiency and aberrant DNA rearrangements due to a hypomorphic RAG1 mutation. Blood 113:2965–2975. https://doi.org/10.1182/blood-2008-07-165167
28. Murphy S, Hayward A, Troup G, Devor E, Coon T (1980) Gene enrichment in an American Indian population: an excess of severe combined immunodeficiency disease. Lancet 2:502–505. https://doi.org/10.1016/s0140-6736(80)91833-4
29. Volk T, Pannicke U, Reisli I, Bulashevska A, Ritter J, Björkman A et al (2015) DCLRE1C (ARTEMIS) mutations causing phenotypes ranging from atypical severe combined immunodeficiency to mere antibody deficiency. Hum Mol Genet 24:7361–7372. https://doi.org/10.1093/hmg/ddv437
30. Pannicke U, Hönig M, Hess I, Friesen C, Holzmann K, Rump EM et al (2009) Reticular dysgenesis (aleukocytosis) is caused by mutations in the gene encoding mitochondrial adenylate kinase 2. Nat Genet 41:101–105. https://doi.org/10.1038/ng.265
31. Dzeja P, Terzic A (2009) Adenylate kinase and AMP signaling networks: metabolic monitoring, signal communication and body energy sensing. Int J Mol Sci 10:1729–1772. https://doi.org/10.3390/ijms10041729
32. Lagresle-Peyrou C, Six EM, Picard C, Rieux-Laucat F, Michel V, Ditadi A et al (2009) Human adenylate kinase 2 deficiency causes a profound hematopoietic defect associated with sensorineural deafness. Nat Genet 41:106–111. https://doi.org/10.1038/ng.278
33. Conway EJ, Cooke R (1939) The deaminases of adenosine and adenylic acid in blood and tissues. Biochem J 33:479–492. https://doi.org/10.1042/bj0330479
34. Cristalli G, Costanzi S, Lambertucci C, Lupidi G, Vittori S, Volpini R et al (2001) Adenosine deaminase: functional implications and different classes of inhibitors. Med Res Rev 21:105–128. https://doi.org/10.1002/1098-1128(200103)21:2<105::aid-med1002>3.0.co;2-u

35. Kwan A, Abraham RS, Currier R, Brower A, Andruszewski K, Abbott JK et al (2014) Newborn screening for severe combined immunodeficiency in 11 screening programs in the United States. JAMA 312:729–738. https://doi.org/10.1001/jama.2014.9132
36. Bradford KL, Moretti FA, Carbonaro-Sarracino DA, Gaspar HB, Kohn DB (2017) Adenosine deaminase (ADA)-deficient severe combined immune deficiency (SCID): molecular pathogenesis and clinical manifestations. J Clin Immunol 37:626–637. https://doi.org/10.1007/s10875-017-0433-3
37. Blackburn MR, Kellems RE (2005) Adenosine deaminase deficiency: metabolic basis of immune deficiency and pulmonary inflammation. Adv Immunol 86:1–41. https://doi.org/10.1016/S0065-2776(04)86001-2
38. Gaspar HB, Aiuti A, Porta F, Candotti F, Hershfield MS, Notarangelo LD (2009) How I treat ADA deficiency. Blood 114:3524–3532. https://doi.org/10.1182/blood-2009-06-189209
39. Flinn AM, Gennery AR (2018) Adenosine deaminase deficiency: a review. Orphanet J Rare Dis 13:65. https://doi.org/10.1186/s13023-018-0807-5
40. Andrews LG, Markert ML (1992) Exon skipping in purine nucleoside phosphorylase mRNA processing leading to severe immunodeficiency. J Biol Chem 267:7834–7838
41. Aust MR, Andrews LG, Barrett MJ, Norby-Slycord CJ, Markert ML (1992) Molecular analysis of mutations in a patient with purine nucleoside phosphorylase deficiency. Am J Hum Genet 51:763–772
42. Williams SR, Gekeler V, McIvor RS, Martin DW (1987) A human purine nucleoside phosphorylase deficiency caused by a single base change. J Biol Chem 262:2332–2338
43. Markert ML, Finkel BD, McLaughlin TM, Watson TJ, Collard HR, McMahon CP et al (1997) Mutations in purine nucleoside phosphorylase deficiency. Hum Mutat 9:118–121. https://doi.org/10.1002/(SICI)1098-1004(1997)9:2<118::AID-HUMU3>3.0.CO;2-5
44. Markert ML (1991) Purine nucleoside phosphorylase deficiency. Immunodefic Rev 3:45–81
45. Biggs CM, Haddad E, Issekutz TB, Roifman CM, Turvey SE (2017) Newborn screening for severe combined immunodeficiency: a primer for clinicians. CMAJ 189:E1551–E1557. https://doi.org/10.1503/cmaj.170561
46. Mazzolari E, de Martiis D, Forino C, Lanfranchi A, Giliani S, Marzollo R et al (2009) Single-center analysis of long-term outcome after hematopoietic cell transplantation in children with congenital severe T cell immunodeficiency. Immunol Res 44:4–17. https://doi.org/10.1007/s12026-008-8022-4
47. Neven B, Leroy S, Decaluwe H, Le Deist F, Picard C, Moshous D et al (2009) Long-term outcome after hematopoietic stem cell transplantation of a single-center cohort of 90 patients with severe combined immunodeficiency. Blood 113:4114–4124. https://doi.org/10.1182/blood-2008-09-177923
48. Railey MD, Lokhnygina Y, Buckley RH (2009) Long-term clinical outcome of patients with severe combined immunodeficiency who received related donor bone marrow transplants without pretransplant chemotherapy or post-transplant GVHD prophylaxis. J Pediatr 155:834–840.e1. https://doi.org/10.1016/j.jpeds.2009.07.049
49. Gennery AR, Slatter MA, Grandin L, Taupin P, Cant AJ, Veys P et al (2010) Transplantation of hematopoietic stem cells and long-term survival for primary immunodeficiencies in Europe: entering a new century, do we do better? J Allergy Clin Immunol 126:602–610.e1–11. https://doi.org/10.1016/j.jaci.2010.06.015
50. Dvorak CC, Cowan MJ, Logan BR, Notarangelo LD, Griffith LM, Puck JM et al (2013) The natural history of children with severe combined immunodeficiency: baseline features of the first fifty patients of the primary immune deficiency treatment consortium prospective study 6901. J Clin Immunol 33:1156–1164. https://doi.org/10.1007/s10875-013-9917-y
51. Heimall J, Logan BR, Cowan MJ, Notarangelo LD, Griffith LM, Puck JM et al (2017) Immune reconstitution and survival of 100 SCID patients post-hematopoietic cell transplant: a PIDTC natural history study. Blood 130:2718–2727. https://doi.org/10.1182/blood-2017-05-781849
52. Pai SY, Logan BR, Griffith LM, Buckley RH, Parrott RE, Dvorak CC et al (2014) Transplantation outcomes for severe combined immunodeficiency, 2000–2009. N Engl J Med 371:434–446. https://doi.org/10.1056/NEJMoa1401177

53. Friedrich W, Hönig M (2010) HLA-haploidentical donor transplantation in severe combined immunodeficiency. Immunol Allergy Clin N Am 30:31–44. https://doi.org/10.1016/j.iac.2009.11.004
54. Haddad E, Logan BR, Griffith LM, Buckley RH, Parrott RE, Prockop SE et al (2018) SCID genotype and 6-month posttransplant CD4 count predict survival and immune recovery. Blood 132:1737–1749. https://doi.org/10.1182/blood-2018-03-840702
55. Gavrilova T (2019) Considerations for hematopoietic stem cell transplantation in primary immunodeficiency disorders. World J Transplant 9:48–57. https://doi.org/10.5500/wjt.v9.i3.48
56. Lum SH, Hoenig M, Gennery AR, Slatter MA (2019) Conditioning regimens for hematopoietic cell transplantation in primary immunodeficiency. Curr Allergy Asthma Rep 19:52. https://doi.org/10.1007/s11882-019-0883-1
57. Cavazzana M, Six E, Lagresle-Peyrou C, André-Schmutz I, Hacein-Bey-Abina S (2016) Gene therapy for X-linked severe combined immunodeficiency: where do we stand? Hum Gene Ther 27:108–116. https://doi.org/10.1089/hum.2015.137
58. Booth C, Gaspar HB (2009) Pegademase bovine (PEG-ADA) for the treatment of infants and children with severe combined immunodeficiency (SCID). Biologics 3:349–358
59. Weinberg K, Hershfield MS, Bastian J, Kohn DB, Sender L, Parkman R et al (1993) T lymphocyte ontogeny in adenosine deaminase-deficient severe combined immune deficiency after treatment with polyethylene glycol-modified adenosine deaminase. J Clin Invest 92:596–602. https://doi.org/10.1172/JCI116626
60. Chan B, Wara D, Bastian J, Hershfield MS, Bohnsack J, Azen CG et al (2005) Long-term efficacy of enzyme replacement therapy for adenosine deaminase (ADA)-deficient severe combined immunodeficiency (SCID). Clin Immunol 117:133–143. https://doi.org/10.1016/j.clim.2005.07.006

Late-Onset and Hypomorphic Presentation of Severe Combined Immune Deficiency

6

Lorenzo Salvati, Boaz Palterer, and Lorenzo Cosmi

Those who have a keen eye, find what they seek even with their eyes closed.

Chi ha occhio, trova quel che cerca anche a occhi chiusi.

In "Marcovaldo" book (1963) by Italo Calvino

6.1 Introduction

Typically, severe combined immunodeficiency (SCID) manifests early in infancy, becoming apparent within the first few months of life [1, 2]. Infants with SCID often exhibit a range of debilitating symptoms, including severe infections caused by opportunistic pathogens, failure to thrive, and other life-threatening complications [1]. If left untreated, SCID follows an unremitting course with fatal outcome before 1 year of age [1, 3]. However, SCID can also present in milder or late-onset forms, broadening the spectrum of clinical presentations that can be observed. These less severe manifestations encompass conditions such as "leaky"/atypical SCID and late-onset combined immunodeficiency (LOCID). In contrast to typical SCID, patients are diagnosed as having leaky (also known as atypical or hypomorphic) SCID when they show less profoundly impaired autologous T-cell differentiation [4]. This leaky phenotype was originally described in some adult SCID mice that could produce detectable serum immunoglobulins and reject skin allografts [5–7]. Table 6.1 presents the Primary Immune Deficiency Treatment Consortium (PIDTC)

L. Salvati · L. Cosmi (✉)
Department of Experimental and Clinical Medicine, University of Florence, Florence, Italy
e-mail: lorenzo.salvati@unifi.it; lorenzo.cosmi@unifi.it

B. Palterer
Boston Children's Hospital, Boston, MA, USA
e-mail: boaz.palterer@unifi.it

M. M. D'Elios (ed.), *Severe Combined Immunodeficiency*, Rare Diseases of the Immune System, https://doi.org/10.1007/978-3-031-78864-2_6

Table 6.1 The Primary Immune Deficiency Treatment Consortium (PIDTC) 2022 definitions for typical and leaky/atypical SCID (from [4])

SCID subtype	Diagnosis requires	Criterion 1	Criterion 2	Criterion 3	Criterion 4
Typical SCID (very low autologous T cells)	Criteria 1 + 2 *OR* Criteria 1 + 3 *OR* Criterion 4	Very low T cells ($<0.05 \times 10^9$/L)[a]	Pathogenic gene variant(s)[b]	No alternate explanation for low T-cell count[c] *AND, EITHER*: Undetectable or low TRECs[d] *OR* <20% of CD4+ T cells have naïve cell surface markers[e]	Presence of TME[f]
Leaky/atypical SCID (low T cells)	Criteria 1 + 2 + 4 *OR* Criteria 1 + 3 + 4	*Two or more of*: • Low T-cell number for age ($0.05–1.0 \times 10^9$/L)[g] • Oligoclonal T cells[h] • Abnormal TRECs *OR* <20% of CD4+ T cells are naïve	Pathogenic gene variant(s)[b]	Reduced proliferation[i]	Does not have: • Other SCID subtype • CID with known genotype • Thymic disorder • Other disorder with low T-cell numbers[j]

[a] T-cell subset determination (with naïve/memory phenotyping) should be repeated at least once, with the second test used as the criterion value. In patients with an identified pathogenic variant, the interval between tests must be at least 1 week; however, in patients without an identified pathogenic gene variant, the T-cell number must remain $<0.05 \times 10^9$/L for at least 8 weeks to qualify as typical SCID due to the potential for spontaneous improvement, with a shorter interval only if urgent hematopoietic cell transplant is required before 8 weeks

[b] Pathogenic variant(s) identified in a gene whose product is known to be essential for T-cell development

[c] Alternate explanations for low T-cell counts include those listed in Criterion 4 of leaky/atypical SCID

[d] Number of TRECs below the normal cutoff, or cycle threshold value above the normal cutoff defined as consistent with SCID by performing laboratory

[e] Naïve T cells should be measured via CD3/CD4/CD45RA, or with additional naïve markers

[f] Transplacentally acquired maternal engraftment; best performed by DNA analysis, such as with short tandem repeats, from whole blood or CD3-separated cells, with any level of detection considered positive. Documented TME classifies patients as typical SCID; TME testing is strongly recommended for patients considered to possibly have leaky/atypical SCID

[g] Low T-cell numbers for age defined as $<0.6 \times 10^9$/L (any age), $<0.8 \times 10^9$/L if aged 2–4 years, or $<1.0 \times 10^9$/L if younger than 2 years

[h] Oligoclonal T cells as defined by laboratory performing testing, for example, <5 peaks in ≥4 T-cell receptor (TCR) Vbeta families on spectra typing, evidence of expansion of ≥2 TCR Vbeta families to >2 × the upper limit of normal for those families, or low Shannon [H] entropy index on high-throughput sequencing of TCR Vbeta variable regions

[i] Reduced proliferation is defined as a proliferative response to PHA, anti-CD3, or anti-CD3/CD28 <50% lower limit of reference range for laboratory

[j] Combined immunodeficiency (including single-gene and syndromic disorders of T-cell development), disorders of thymic stromal cell development, idiopathic T-cell lymphopenia, or secondary T-cell lymphopenia

2022 criteria for SCID classification [4]. These revised definitions have demonstrated superior accuracy in characterizing leaky/atypical SCID when compared to the previously established PIDTC 2014 definitions [8, 9].

Leaky/atypical SCID refers to patients with partial defects in T-cell numbers, diversity, and maturity, due to hypomorphic or "leaky" pathogenic variant(s) in the same gene(s) causing typical SCID (termed "leaky SCID"), or arising from defects that have not yet been identified (termed "atypical SCID") [4]. The 6901 Prospective Study conducted by the PIDTC in the Unites States and Canada revealed that nearly 90% of patients diagnosed with leaky/atypical SCID have an identified pathogenic gene variant, leading them to be classified as having leaky SCID [10]. The most commonly implicated genes in these cases included RAG1, RAG2, IL2RG, ADA, RMRP, ZAP70, AK2, and JAK3 [10].

In the context of common variable immunodeficiency (CVID), patients who experience opportunistic infections and/or have a profound T-cell defect (as defined as CD4+ T-cell count $<0.2 \times 10^9$ cells/L or naïve CD4+ T-cell count $<0.02 \times 10^9$ cells/L) are defined as having LOCID [11, 12].

The recognition of these alternative presentations is progressively being acknowledged in the field of inborn errors of immunity (IEI) and is actively expanding the spectrum of IEI. One of the consequences of the adoption of next-generation sequencing technologies and the use of large gene panels or unbiased approaches such as whole-exome sequencing and whole-genome sequencing is the serendipitous discovery of patients with variants in classically SCID genes but presenting with an array of clinical phenotypes ranging from leaky SCID and LOCID, to milder defects such as CVID.

IEI are characterized by a remarkable genetic heterogeneity, meaning that the same clinical phenotype can arise from variants in many genes [13]. This contributes to the complexity of those conditions and their diagnostic challenges. Conversely, there is emerging evidence of genetic pleiotropism in IEI, meaning that variants within a single gene can generate different clinical phenotypes [13]. Hence, distinct genetic alterations in the same gene can result in varied manifestations of SCID, further highlighting the intricate relationship between genetics and the clinical phenotype.

6.2 Mechanisms

The main mechanisms responsible for leaky/atypical presentations of SCID are hypomorphic variants, mosaicism, and somatic reversion.

Genetic variants can be classified according to their effect on the produced protein in synonymous, missense, nonsense, splicing, or frameshift [14]. In general, insertion/deletion leading to frameshifts or nonsense variants leading to truncated protein causes a loss-of-function (LOF). Missense variants are single nucleotide variants, leading to a single aminoacidic substitution. The effects on protein function of missense variants are less predictable and can range anywhere from LOF, to variably reduced activity (hypomorphic), to increased or new activity (gain-of-function).

Hypomorphic variants have been identified in several SCID genes and may give rise to milder or later-onset forms of the disease, exhibiting variable clinical phenotypes compared to the classical form.

Mosaicism occurs when two or more populations of cells with different genetic compositions are present in the same individual [15]. This phenomenon manifests as the affected genetic variant being confined to specific lineages of cells, resulting in varying degrees of immune dysfunction [16]. Mosaicism can result from DNA mutations, epigenetic alterations, chromosomal abnormalities, and the spontaneous reversion of inherited mutations. Somatic reversion occurs when a spontaneous genetic correction takes place in somatic cells, leading to the restoration of normal gene function. This phenomenon has been particularly observed in IL2RG deficiency and Wiskott-Aldrich syndrome. Individuals with somatic reversion may exhibit partial restoration of immune function, resulting in milder clinical manifestations compared to the classical presentation of the disease. Somatic reversion can occur through various mechanisms, such as spontaneous DNA repair or recombination events, leading to the emergence of cells with corrected genetic sequences [17, 18].

In 1996, an atypical form of X-linked SCID—characterized by the presence of circulating mature T cells—was reported, where a partial reversion of γc gene mutation occurred in lymphocyte progenitor cells, leading to the emergence of partially functional lymphocyte clones [19]. The existence of milder phenotypes of X-SCID due to IL2RG reversion events must be taken into consideration, as this form of presentation can delay the diagnosis [20–25].

In 1993, low lymphocyte and erythrocyte adenosine deaminase (ADA) activity together with accumulated deoxyadenosine triphosphate (dATP) in erythrocytes and deoxyadenosine in urine was described in two adult sisters with chronic pulmonary disease and recurrent bacterial, viral, and fungal infections [26]. Adult presentation of adenosine deaminase deficiency results from partial deaminase activity of variant protein [27], but also somatic mosaicism has been reported [28, 29].

RAG deficiency is arguably the best understood example of genetic pleiotropism in SCID. There is a direct correlation between the recombination activity of RAG variants, TCR repertoire diversity, and clinical phenotype [30]. While null mutations in the RAG genes lead to T−B−SCID, it has been shown that hypomorphic RAG mutations—due to different levels of recombination activity of the mutant RAG proteins—are associated with defects in central and peripheral tolerance, resulting in immune dysregulation [31].

The immune impairment of DNA ligase IV deficiency can vary from radiosensitive SCID to milder forms due to hypomorphic mutations [32–34].

6.3 Diagnostic Challenges

Late-onset and hypomorphic presentations of SCID pose significant challenges for diagnosis. Routine immunological tests can yield borderline results, making it difficult to establish a clear-cut diagnosis. Furthermore, functional tests designed to assess immune system functionality can be hard to interpret accurately, adding to the complexity of the diagnostic process. Another challenge arises in the context of newborn screening, where the sensitivity to detect atypical SCID may be reduced or on the other side asymptomatic children can be identified [35]. The reduction in sensitivity can potentially lead to missed or delayed identification of affected infants, further complicating timely intervention. On the contrary, the identification of asymptomatic infants leads to early diagnosis and question potential treatments before overt phenotype eventually arises.

From a genetic perspective, the presence of hypomorphic variants adds another layer of complexity to the diagnostic challenge. Hypomorphic variants often fall into the category of variants of uncertain significance (VUS). Distinguishing the clinical implications and severity of hypomorphic variants is generally more challenging compared to null variants that completely abolish gene function [36]. In fact, hypomorphic variants can cause a diverse spectrum of phenotypes, ranging from severe to mild or no apparent clinical effects. In the latter instances, the phenomenon is called incomplete penetrance, meaning that individuals carrying the variant may not exhibit any symptoms or may have milder symptoms than expected [37]. The degree of the reduction in gene function can significantly influence the resulting phenotype. Nonetheless, even among individuals with the same hypomorphic variant, the severity and presentation of the condition can vary. This variability can be influenced by genetic modifiers, environmental factors, or other variables. In contrast to null variants that typically show a clear loss of function that can be detected using various laboratory assays, hypomorphic variants often require more sophisticated and highly sensitive assays to detect subtle changes in gene function or protein activity [38].

Furthermore, somatic reversion and mosaicism can easily go undetected using standard sequencing technologies due to their low allele fraction and the limitations of the sequencing methods [39]. Standard sequencing technologies often have a detection limit of around 5–10% variant allele frequency. Mutations occurring at lower frequencies may be below this threshold and, consequently, remain undetected. Variant calling algorithms used in standard sequencing data analysis are optimized to identify common genetic variants and may not be sensitive enough to detect rare or low-frequency variants. These algorithms often rely on a minimum threshold for supporting reads at a variant site to reduce false positives, but this threshold can lead to the omission of true low-frequency mutations. Standard sequencing platforms typically generate a fixed depth of coverage for each position in the genome. While this depth is usually sufficient for identifying germline mutations or common somatic mutations, it may not provide adequate coverage to confidently identify rare somatic variants. Sequencing errors can occur during the sample preparation, sequencing, and base calling steps, leading to false positive variant calls, especially when dealing with low-frequency variants. The presence of sequencing errors at low allele fractions can be difficult to distinguish from true somatic mutations. Somatic reversion and mosaicism are more likely to be obscured if the sample contains a mixture of cells, including both wild-type and mutant cells. In such cases, the signal from the low-frequency variant may be overwhelmed by the dominant wild-type signal. To address these challenges and improve detection, ultra-deep sequencing, single-cell sequencing, or targeted sequencing can be used

[40]. Increasing the depth of sequencing to hundreds or thousands of reads per position can enhance sensitivity and facilitate the detection of low-frequency variants. Single-cell sequencing enables the analysis of individual cells, allowing for the identification of mosaic mutations present in only a small fraction of cells. Finally, focusing on specific genomic regions of interest can increase the depth of coverage for those regions, improving the likelihood of detecting low-frequency variants.

The interpretation of a genetic test is particularly challenging when the variant is identified for the first time in a single patient. One of the valuable resources in this field is the Clinical Genome Resource (ClinGen) [41]. This comprehensive resource supported by the National Institute of Health (NIH) collects detailed phenotypic and clinical information on genetic variants across the entire genome. By aggregating and analyzing this data, ClinGen develops consensus approaches to identify the clinical relevance of these variants [42]. The information gathered is then disseminated to researchers and clinicians, providing a robust foundation for improving diagnostic accuracy and treatment strategies [41].

6.4 Therapeutic Approaches

The transition from traditional clinical classifications (SCID) to the era of molecular diagnostics (specific genetic alterations) has marked a paradigm shift in the therapeutic approach [43]. Patients with molecular diagnosis that do not fit the clinical label are increasingly being reported. This is challenging because historically treatments were dictated by the clinical phenotype: SCID traditionally warrants hematopoietic stem cell transplantation (HSCT). The primary and life-saving therapeutic approach for most SCID is indeed HSCT, which offers the potential for immune reconstitution and long-term survival [44]. However, the success and outcomes of HSCT can vary depending on several factors, including the specific type and severity of SCID, as well as the timing and conditioning [45–48]. Population-based newborn screening leads to prompt HSCT at an earlier age and more often without previous history of infections, resulting into improved outcome [49].

In addition, specific conditions now benefit from tailored therapeutic interventions shaped by their genetic etiology. Notably, gene therapy in ADA deficiency, IL2RG deficiency, and Artemis deficiency leads to immune reconstitution in most patients [50–55]. By correcting the genetic defect responsible for the immune system dysfunction, gene therapy offers the possibility of restoring normal immune function and improving patient outcomes [56]. In addition to therapeutical interventions, genetic counseling and patient and family support play crucial roles in managing SCID.

6.5 Conclusion

"Those who have an eye, find what they seek even with their eyes closed." The current challenges in diagnosing atypical presentations of SCID require a keen eye and persistence, similar to *Marcovaldo's* wandering around a dry fountain in a summer night and his instinctive realization that an artificial basin must have a faucet [57]. The essence lies in discovering the faucet where conventional expectations wouldn't place it. Specifically, an increasing number of individuals with molecular diagnoses that deviate from the anticipated clinical labels are uncovered, fundamentally reshaping treatment paradigms towards targeted and individualized approaches.

References

1. Fischer A, Notarangelo LD, Neven B, Cavazzana M, Puck JM (2015) Severe combined immunodeficiencies and related disorders. Nat Rev Dis Primers 1:15061. https://doi.org/10.1038/nrdp.2015.61
2. Fischer A (1992) Severe combined immunodeficiencies. Immunodefic Rev 3(2):83–100
3. de Pagter AP, Bredius RG, Kuijpers TW, Tramper J, van der Burg M, van Montfrans J, Driessen GJ, Dutch Working Party for Immunodeficiencies (2015) Overview of 15-year severe combined immunodeficiency in The Netherlands: towards newborn blood spot screening. Eur J Pediatr 174(9):1183–1188. https://doi.org/10.1007/s00431-015-2518-4. Epub 2015 Apr 1
4. Dvorak CC, Haddad E, Heimall J, Dunn E, Buckley RH, Kohn DB, Cowan MJ, Pai SY, Griffith LM, Cuvelier GDE, Eissa H, Shah AJ, O'Reilly RJ, Pulsipher MA, Wright NAM, Abraham RS, Satter LF, Notarangelo LD, Puck JM (2023) The diagnosis of severe combined immunodeficiency (SCID): The Primary Immune Deficiency Treatment Consortium (PIDTC) 2022 Definitions. J Allergy Clin Immunol 151(2):539–546. https://doi.org/10.1016/j.jaci.2022.10.022. Epub 2022 Nov 28
5. Carroll AM, Hardy RR, Petrini J, Bosma MJ (1989) T cell leakiness in SCID mice. Curr Top Microbiol Immunol 152:117–123. https://doi.org/10.1007/978-3-642-74974-2_15
6. Bosma GC, Fried M, Custer RP, Carroll A, Gibson DM, Bosma MJ (1988) Evidence of functional lymphocytes in some (leaky) SCID mice. J Exp Med 167(3):1016–1033. https://doi.org/10.1084/jem.167.3.1016
7. Carroll AM, Bosma MJ (1988) Detection and characterization of functional T cells in mice with severe combined immune deficiency. Eur J Immunol 18(12):1965–1971. https://doi.org/10.1002/eji.1830181215
8. Dvorak CC, Haddad E, Heimall J, Dunn E, Cowan MJ, Pai SY, Kapoor N, Satter LF, Buckley RH, O'Reilly RJ, Chandra S, Bednarski JJ, Williams O, Rayes A, Moore TB, Ebens CL, Davila Saldana BJ, Petrovic A, Chellapandian D, Cuvelier GDE, Vander Lugt MT, Caywood EH, Chandrakasan S, Eissa H, Goldman FD, Shereck E, Aquino VM, Desantes KB, Madden LM, Miller HK, Yu L, Broglie L, Gillio A, Shah AJ, Knutsen AP, Andolina JP, Joshi AY, Szabolcs P, Kapadia M, Martinez CA, Parrot RE, Sullivan KE, Prockop SE, Abraham RS, Thakar MS, Leiding JW, Kohn DB, Pulsipher MA, Griffith LM, Notarangelo LD, Puck JM (2023) The diagnosis of severe combined immunodeficiency: implementation of the PIDTC 2022 Definitions. J Allergy Clin Immunol 151(2):547–555.e5. https://doi.org/10.1016/j.jaci.2022.10.021. Epub 2022 Nov 28
9. Shearer WT, Dunn E, Notarangelo LD, Dvorak CC, Puck JM, Logan BR, Griffith LM, Kohn DB, O'Reilly RJ, Fleisher TA, Pai SY, Martinez CA, Buckley RH, Cowan MJ (2014) Establishing diagnostic criteria for severe combined immunodeficiency disease (SCID), leaky SCID, and Omenn syndrome: the Primary Immune Deficiency Treatment Consortium experience. J Allergy Clin Immunol 133(4):1092–1098. https://doi.org/10.1016/j.jaci.2013.09.044. Epub 2013 Nov 28
10. Dvorak CC, Haddad E, Buckley RH, Cowan MJ, Logan B, Griffith LM, Kohn DB, Pai SY, Notarangelo L, Shearer W, Prockop S, Kapoor N, Heimall J, Chaudhury S, Shyr D, Chandra S, Cuvelier G, Moore T, Shenoy S, Goldman F, Smith AR, Sunkersett G, Vander Lugt M, Caywood E, Quigg T, Torgerson T, Chandrakasan S, Craddock J, Dávila Saldaña BJ, Gillio A, Shereck E, Aquino V, DeSantes K, Knutsen A, Thakar M, Yu L, Puck JM (2019) The genetic

landscape of severe combined immunodeficiency in the United States and Canada in the current era (2010–2018). J Allergy Clin Immunol 143(1):405–407. https://doi.org/10.1016/j.jaci.2018.08.027. Epub 2018 Sep 5

11. Malphettes M, Gérard L, Carmagnat M, Mouillot G, Vince N, Boutboul D, Bérezné A, Nove-Josserand R, Lemoing V, Tetu L, Viallard JF, Bonnotte B, Pavic M, Haroche J, Larroche C, Brouet JC, Fermand JP, Rabian C, Fieschi C, Oksenhendler E, DEFI Study Group (2009) Late-onset combined immune deficiency: a subset of common variable immunodeficiency with severe T cell defect. Clin Infect Dis 49(9):1329–1338. https://doi.org/10.1086/606059
12. Bertinchamp R, Gérard L, Boutboul D, Malphettes M, Fieschi C, Oksenhendler E, DEFI study group (2016) Exclusion of patients with a severe T-cell defect improves the definition of common variable immunodeficiency. J Allergy Clin Immunol Pract 4(6):1147–1157. https://doi.org/10.1016/j.jaip.2016.07.002. Epub 2016 Aug 10
13. Notarangelo LD, Bacchetta R, Casanova JL, Su HC (2020) Human inborn errors of immunity: an expanding universe. Sci Immunol 5(49):eabb1662. https://doi.org/10.1126/sciimmunol.abb1662
14. Richards S, Aziz N, Bale S, Bick D, Das S, Gastier-Foster J, Grody WW, Hegde M, Lyon E, Spector E, Voelkerding K, Rehm HL, ACMG Laboratory Quality Assurance Committee (2015) Standards and guidelines for the interpretation of sequence variants: a joint consensus recommendation of the American College of Medical Genetics and Genomics and the Association for Molecular Pathology. Genet Med 17(5):405–424. https://doi.org/10.1038/gim.2015.30. Epub 2015 Mar 5
15. Miyazawa H, Wada T (2021) Reversion mosaicism in primary immunodeficiency diseases. Front Immunol 12:783022. https://doi.org/10.3389/fimmu.2021.783022
16. Mensa-Vilaró A, Bravo García-Morato M, de la Calle-Martin O, Franco-Jarava C, Martínez-Saavedra MT, González-Granado LI, González-Roca E, Fuster JL, Alsina L, Mutchinick OM, Balderrama-Rodríguez A, Ramos E, Modesto C, Mesa-Del-Castillo P, Ortego-Centeno N, Clemente D, Souto A, Palmou N, Remesal A, Leslie KS, Gómez de la Fuente E, Yadira Bravo Gallego L, Campistol JM, Dhouib NG, Bejaoui M, Dutra LA, Terreri MT, Mosquera C, González T, Cañellas J, García-Ruiz de Morales JM, Wouters CH, Bosque MT, Cham WT, Jiménez-Treviño S, de Inocencio J, Bloomfield M, Pérez de Diego R, Martínez-Pomar N, Rodríguez-Pena R, González-Santesteban C, Soler-Palacín P, Casals F, Yagüe J, Allende LM, Rodríguez-Gallego JC, Colobran R, Martínez-Martínez L, López-Granados E, Aróstegui JI (2019) Unexpected relevant role of gene mosaicism in patients with primary immunodeficiency diseases. J Allergy Clin Immunol 143(1):359–368. https://doi.org/10.1016/j.jaci.2018.09.009. Epub 2018 Sep 29
17. Davis BR, Candotti F (2009) Revertant somatic mosaicism in the Wiskott-Aldrich syndrome. Immunol Res 44(1–3):127–131. https://doi.org/10.1007/s12026-008-8091-4
18. Wada T, Schurman SH, Otsu M, Garabedian EK, Ochs HD, Nelson DL, Candotti F (2001) Somatic mosaicism in Wiskott–Aldrich syndrome suggests in vivo reversion by a DNA slippage mechanism. Proc Natl Acad Sci USA 98(15):8697–8702. https://doi.org/10.1073/pnas.151260498. Epub 2001 Jul 10
19. Stephan V, Wahn V, Le Deist F, Dirksen U, Broker B, Müller-Fleckenstein I, Horneff G, Schroten H, Fischer A, de Saint Basile G (1996) Atypical X-linked severe combined immunodeficiency due to possible spontaneous reversion of the genetic defect in T cells. N Engl J Med 335(21):1563–1567. https://doi.org/10.1056/NEJM199611213352104
20. Hsu AP, Pittaluga S, Martinez B, Rump AP, Raffeld M, Uzel G, Puck JM, Freeman AF, Holland SM (2015) IL2RG reversion event in a common lymphoid progenitor leads to delayed diagnosis and milder phenotype. J Clin Immunol 35(5):449–453. https://doi.org/10.1007/s10875-015-0174-0. Epub 2015 Jun 17
21. Okuno Y, Hoshino A, Muramatsu H, Kawashima N, Wang X, Yoshida K, Wada T, Gunji M, Toma T, Kato T, Shiraishi Y, Iwata A, Hori T, Kitoh T, Chiba K, Tanaka H, Sanada M, Takahashi Y, Nonoyama S, Ito M, Miyano S, Ogawa S, Kojima S, Kanegane H (2015) Late-onset combined immunodeficiency with a novel IL2RG mutation and probable revertant somatic mosa-

icism. J Clin Immunol 35(7):610–614. https://doi.org/10.1007/s10875-015-0202-0. Epub 2015 Sep 26
22. Speckmann C, Pannicke U, Wiech E, Schwarz K, Fisch P, Friedrich W, Niehues T, Gilmour K, Buiting K, Schlesier M, Eibel H, Rohr J, Superti-Furga A, Gross-Wieltsch U, Ehl S (2008) Clinical and immunologic consequences of a somatic reversion in a patient with X-linked severe combined immunodeficiency. Blood 112(10):4090–4097. https://doi.org/10.1182/blood-2008-04-153361. Epub 2008 Aug 26
23. Wada T, Yasui M, Toma T, Nakayama Y, Nishida M, Shimizu M, Okajima M, Kasahara Y, Koizumi S, Inoue M, Kawa K, Yachie A (2008) Detection of T lymphocytes with a second-site mutation in skin lesions of atypical X-linked severe combined immunodeficiency mimicking Omenn syndrome. Blood 112(5):1872–1875. https://doi.org/10.1182/blood-2008-04-149708. Epub 2008 Jun 16
24. Kawai T, Saito M, Nishikomori R, Yasumi T, Izawa K, Murakami T, Okamoto S, Mori Y, Nakagawa N, Imai K, Nonoyama S, Wada T, Yachie A, Ohmori K, Nakahata T, Heike T (2012) Multiple reversions of an IL2RG mutation restore T cell function in an X-linked severe combined immunodeficiency patient. J Clin Immunol 32(4):690–697. https://doi.org/10.1007/s10875-012-9684-1. Epub 2012 Mar 30
25. Kuijpers TW, van Leeuwen EM, Barendregt BH, Klarenbeek P, aan de Kerk DJ, Baars PA, Jansen MH, de Vries N, van Lier RA, van der Burg M (2013) A reversion of an IL2RG mutation in combined immunodeficiency providing competitive advantage to the majority of CD8+ T cells. Haematologica 98(7):1030–1038. https://doi.org/10.3324/haematol.2012.077511. Epub 2013 Feb 12
26. Shovlin CL, Hughes JM, Simmonds HA, Fairbanks L, Deacock S, Lechler R, Roberts I, Webster AD (1993) Adult presentation of adenosine deaminase deficiency. Lancet 341(8858):1471. https://doi.org/10.1016/0140-6736(93)90910-9
27. Ozsahin H, Arredondo-Vega FX, Santisteban I, Fuhrer H, Tuchschmid P, Jochum W, Aguzzi A, Lederman HM, Fleischman A, Winkelstein JA, Seger RA, Hershfield MS (1997) Adenosine deaminase deficiency in adults. Blood 89(8):2849–2855
28. Hirschhorn R, Yang DR, Israni A, Huie ML, Ownby DR (1994) Somatic mosaicism for a newly identified splice-site mutation in a patient with adenosine deaminase-deficient immunodeficiency and spontaneous clinical recovery. Am J Hum Genet 55(1):59–68
29. Hirschhorn R, Yang DR, Puck JM, Huie ML, Jiang CK, Kurlandsky LE (1996) Spontaneous in vivo reversion to normal of an inherited mutation in a patient with adenosine deaminase deficiency. Nat Genet 13(3):290–295. https://doi.org/10.1038/ng0796-290
30. Bosticardo M, Pala F, Notarangelo LD (2021) RAG deficiencies: recent advances in disease pathogenesis and novel therapeutic approaches. Eur J Immunol 51(5):1028–1038. https://doi.org/10.1002/eji.202048880. Epub 2021 Mar 22
31. Villa A, Notarangelo LD (2019) RAG gene defects at the verge of immunodeficiency and immune dysregulation. Immunol Rev 287(1):73–90. https://doi.org/10.1111/imr.12713
32. Staines Boone AT, Chinn IK, Alaez-Versón C, Yamazaki-Nakashimada MA, Carrillo-Sánchez K, García-Cruz MLH, Poli MC, González Serrano ME, Medina Torres EA, Muzquiz Zermeño D, Forbes LR, Espinosa-Rosales FJ, Espinosa-Padilla SE, Orange JS, Lugo Reyes SO (2019) Failing to make ends meet: the broad clinical spectrum of DNA ligase IV deficiency. Case series and review of the literature. Front Pediatr 6:426. https://doi.org/10.3389/fped.2018.00426
33. van der Burg M, van Veelen LR, Verkaik NS, Wiegant WW, Hartwig NG, Barendregt BH, Brugmans L, Raams A, Jaspers NG, Zdzienicka MZ, van Dongen JJ, van Gent DC (2006) A new type of radiosensitive T−B−NK+ severe combined immunodeficiency caused by a LIG4 mutation. J Clin Invest 116(1):137–145. https://doi.org/10.1172/JCI26121. Epub 2005 Dec 15
34. Cifaldi C, Angelino G, Chiriaco M, Di Cesare S, Claps A, Serafinelli J, Rossi P, Antoccia A, Di Matteo G, Cancrini C, De Villartay JP, Finocchi A (2017 Mar) Late-onset combined immune deficiency due to LIGIV mutations in a 12-year-old patient. Pediatr Allergy Immunol 28(2):203–206. https://doi.org/10.1111/pai.12684
35. Chitty-Lopez M, Westermann-Clark E, Dawson I, Ujhazi B, Csomos K, Dobbs K, Le K, Yamazaki Y, Sadighi Akha AA, Chellapandian D, Oshrine B, Notarangelo LD, Sunkersett

G, Leiding JW, Walter JE (2020) Asymptomatic infant with atypical SCID and novel hypomorphic RAG variant identified by newborn screening: a diagnostic and treatment dilemma. Front Immunol 11:1954. https://doi.org/10.3389/fimmu.2020.01954
36. Chinn IK, Chan AY, Chen K, Chou J, Dorsey MJ, Hajjar J, Jongco AM III, Keller MD, Kobrynski LJ, Kumanovics A, Lawrence MG, Leiding JW, Lugar PL, Orange JS, Patel K, Platt CD, Puck JM, Raje N, Romberg N, Slack MA, Sullivan KE, Tarrant TK, Torgerson TR, Walter JE (2020) Diagnostic interpretation of genetic studies in patients with primary immunodeficiency diseases: a working group report of the Primary Immunodeficiency Diseases Committee of the American Academy of Allergy, Asthma & Immunology. J Allergy Clin Immunol 145(1):46–69. https://doi.org/10.1016/j.jaci.2019.09.009. Epub 2019 Sep 27
37. Cooper DN, Krawczak M, Polychronakos C, Tyler-Smith C, Kehrer-Sawatzki H (2013) Where genotype is not predictive of phenotype: towards an understanding of the molecular basis of reduced penetrance in human inherited disease. Hum Genet 132(10):1077–1130. https://doi.org/10.1007/s00439-013-1331-2. Epub 2013 Jul 3
38. Haque N, Kawai T, Ratnasinghe BD, Wagenknecht JB, Urrutia R, Notarangelo LD, Zimmermann MT (2023) RAG genomic variation causes autoimmune diseases through specific structure-based mechanisms of enzyme dysregulation. iScience 26(10):108040. https://doi.org/10.1016/j.isci.2023.108040
39. Gajecka M (2016) Unrevealed mosaicism in the next-generation sequencing era. Mol Genet Genomics 291(2):513–530. https://doi.org/10.1007/s00438-015-1130-7. Epub 2015 Oct 19
40. Lee K, Abraham RS (2021) Next-generation sequencing for inborn errors of immunity. Hum Immunol 82(11):871–882. https://doi.org/10.1016/j.humimm.2021.02.011. Epub 2021 Mar 11
41. Rehm HL, Berg JS, Brooks LD, Bustamante CD, Evans JP, Landrum MJ, Ledbetter DH, Maglott DR, Martin CL, Nussbaum RL, Plon SE, Ramos EM, Sherry ST, Watson MS, ClinGen (2015) ClinGen—the clinical genome resource. N Engl J Med 372(23):2235–2242. https://doi.org/10.1056/NEJMsr1406261. Epub 2015 May 27
42. Strande NT, Riggs ER, Buchanan AH, Ceyhan-Birsoy O, DiStefano M, Dwight SS, Goldstein J, Ghosh R, Seifert BA, Sneddon TP, Wright MW, Milko LV, Cherry JM, Giovanni MA, Murray MF, O'Daniel JM, Ramos EM, Santani AB, Scott AF, Plon SE, Rehm HL, Martin CL, Berg JS (2017) Evaluating the clinical validity of gene-disease associations: an evidence-based framework developed by the clinical genome resource. Am J Hum Genet 100(6):895–906. https://doi.org/10.1016/j.ajhg.2017.04.015. Epub 2017 May 25
43. Slatter MA, Gennery AR (2022) Advances in the treatment of severe combined immunodeficiency. Clin Immunol 242:109084. https://doi.org/10.1016/j.clim.2022.109084. Epub 2022 Aug 5
44. Haddad E, Hoenig M (2019) Hematopoietic stem cell transplantation for severe combined immunodeficiency (SCID). Front Pediatr 7:481. https://doi.org/10.3389/fped.2019.00481
45. Abd Hamid IJ, Slatter MA, McKendrick F, Pearce MS, Gennery AR (2017) Long-term outcome of hematopoietic stem cell transplantation for IL2RG/JAK3 SCID: a cohort report. Blood 129(15):2198–2201. https://doi.org/10.1182/blood-2016-11-748616. Epub 2017 Feb 16
46. Schuetz C, Neven B, Dvorak CC, Leroy S, Ege MJ, Pannicke U, Schwarz K, Schulz AS, Hoenig M, Sparber-Sauer M, Gatz SA, Denzer C, Blanche S, Moshous D, Picard C, Horn BN, de Villartay JP, Cavazzana M, Debatin KM, Friedrich W, Fischer A, Cowan MJ (2014) SCID patients with ARTEMIS vs RAG deficiencies following HCT: increased risk of late toxicity in ARTEMIS-deficient SCID. Blood 123(2):281–289. https://doi.org/10.1182/blood-2013-01-476432. Epub 2013 Oct 21. Erratum in: Blood. 2018 Dec 6;132(23):2527
47. Ghimenton E, Flinn A, Lum SH, Leahy TR, Nademi Z, Owens S, Williams E, Flood T, Hambleton S, Slatter M, Gennery AR (2022) Hematopoietic cell transplantation for adenosine deaminase severe combined immunodeficiency-improved outcomes in the modern era. J Clin Immunol 42(4):819–826. https://doi.org/10.1007/s10875-022-01238-0. Epub 2022 Mar 15
48. Pai SY, Logan BR, Griffith LM, Buckley RH, Parrott RE, Dvorak CC, Kapoor N, Hanson IC, Filipovich AH, Jyonouchi S, Sullivan KE, Small TN, Burroughs L, Skoda-Smith S, Haight AE, Grizzle A, Pulsipher MA, Chan KW, Fuleihan RL, Haddad E, Loechelt B, Aquino VM, Gillio A, Davis J, Knutsen A, Smith AR, Moore TB, Schroeder ML, Goldman FD, Connelly

JA, Porteus MH, Xiang Q, Shearer WT, Fleisher TA, Kohn DB, Puck JM, Notarangelo LD, Cowan MJ, O'Reilly RJ (2014) Transplantation outcomes for severe combined immunodeficiency, 2000–2009. N Engl J Med 371(5):434–446. https://doi.org/10.1056/NEJMoa1401177

49. Thakar MS, Logan BR, Puck JM, Dunn EA, Buckley RH, Cowan MJ, O'Reilly RJ, Kapoor N, Satter LF, Pai SY, Heimall J, Chandra S, Ebens CL, Chellapandian D, Williams O, Burroughs LM, Saldana BD, Rayes A, Madden LM, Chandrakasan S, Bednarski JJ II, DeSantes KB, Cuvelier GDE, Teira P, Gillio AP, Eissa H, Knutsen AP, Goldman FD, Aquino VM, Shereck EB, Moore TB, Caywood EH, Lugt MTV, Rozmus J, Broglie L, Yu LC, Shah AJ, Andolina JR, Liu X, Parrott RE, Dara J, Prockop S, Martinez CA, Kapadia M, Jyonouchi SC, Sullivan KE, Bleesing JJ, Chaudhury S, Petrovic A, Keller MD, Quigg TC, Parikh S, Shenoy S, Seroogy C, Rubin T, Decaluwe H, Routes JM, Torgerson TR, Leiding JW, Pulsipher MA, Kohn DB, Griffith LM, Haddad E, Dvorak CC, Notarangelo LD (2023) Measuring the effect of newborn screening on survival after haematopoietic cell transplantation for severe combined immunodeficiency: a 36-year longitudinal study from the Primary Immune Deficiency Treatment Consortium. Lancet 402(10396):129–140. https://doi.org/10.1016/S0140-6736(23)00731-6. Epub 2023 Jun 20
50. Aiuti A, Slavin S, Aker M, Ficara F, Deola S, Mortellaro A, Morecki S, Andolfi G, Tabucchi A, Carlucci F, Marinello E, Cattaneo F, Vai S, Servida P, Miniero R, Roncarolo MG, Bordignon C (2002) Correction of ADA-SCID by stem cell gene therapy combined with nonmyeloablative conditioning. Science 296(5577):2410–2413. https://doi.org/10.1126/science.1070104
51. Aiuti A, Cattaneo F, Galimberti S, Benninghoff U, Cassani B, Callegaro L, Scaramuzza S, Andolfi G, Mirolo M, Brigida I, Tabucchi A, Carlucci F, Eibl M, Aker M, Slavin S, Al-Mousa H, Al Ghonaium A, Ferster A, Duppenthaler A, Notarangelo L, Wintergerst U, Buckley RH, Bregni M, Marktel S, Valsecchi MG, Rossi P, Ciceri F, Miniero R, Bordignon C, Roncarolo MG (2009) Gene therapy for immunodeficiency due to adenosine deaminase deficiency. N Engl J Med 360(5):447–458. https://doi.org/10.1056/NEJMoa0805817
52. Gaspar HB, Aiuti A, Porta F, Candotti F, Hershfield MS, Notarangelo LD (2009) How I treat ADA deficiency. Blood 114(17):3524–3532. https://doi.org/10.1182/blood-2009-06-189209. Epub 2009 Jul 28
53. Reinhardt B, Habib O, Shaw KL, Garabedian E, Carbonaro-Sarracino DA, Terrazas D, Fernandez BC, De Oliveira S, Moore TB, Ikeda AK, Engel BC, Podsakoff GM, Hollis RP, Fernandes A, Jackson C, Shupien S, Mishra S, Davila A, Mottahedeh J, Vitomirov A, Meng W, Rosenfeld AM, Roche AM, Hokama P, Reddy S, Everett J, Wang X, Luning Prak ET, Cornetta K, Hershfield MS, Sokolic R, De Ravin SS, Malech HL, Bushman FD, Candotti F, Kohn DB (2021) Long-term outcomes after gene therapy for adenosine deaminase severe combined immune deficiency. Blood 138(15):1304–1316. https://doi.org/10.1182/blood.2020010260
54. Blanco E, Izotova N, Booth C, Thrasher AJ (2020) Immune reconstitution after gene therapy approaches in patients with X-linked severe combined immunodeficiency disease. Front Immunol 11:608653. https://doi.org/10.3389/fimmu.2020.608653
55. Cowan MJ, Yu J, Facchino J, Fraser-Browne C, Sanford U, Kawahara M, Dara J, Long-Boyle J, Oh J, Chan W, Chag S, Broderick L, Chellapandian D, Decaluwe H, Golski C, Hu D, Kuo CY, Miller HK, Petrovic A, Currier R, Hilton JF, Punwani D, Dvorak CC, Malech HL, McIvor RS, Puck JM (2022) Lentiviral gene therapy for Artemis-deficient SCID. N Engl J Med 387(25):2344–2355. https://doi.org/10.1056/NEJMoa2206575
56. Fischer A (2023) Gene therapy for inborn errors of immunity: past, present and future. Nat Rev Immunol 23(6):397–408. https://doi.org/10.1038/s41577-022-00800-6. Epub 2022 Nov 25
57. Italo C (1963) Marcovaldo or the seasons in the city. Mariner Books, Italy

Gut Involvement in Cellular Immunodeficiencies

7

Sofia D'Elios, Marisa Benagiano, Evangelina Asvestopoulou, Mario Milco D'Elios, and Chiara Della Bella

Different factors, as the nature of the immune defect, along with the specific part of the gastrointestinal tract (Fig. 7.1) affected, as well as the type of pathogenic stimuli, ranging from pathogens to allergens, influences the clinical outcomes.

Individuals with primary cellular immunodeficiencies may experience infectious, inflammatory, autoimmune, and malignant symptoms at various levels of the digestive tract.

The gastrointestinal clinical presentation of PID patients may mimic classical gut diseases, as common gastroenteritis, autoimmune or inflammatory diseases like celiac disease or inflammatory bowel disease. The atypical age of symptoms onset or distinctive histology, and a lack of response to conventional treatments may raise suspicion that an underlying immune system defect is occurring.

In such instances, a basic screening involving protein electrophoresis and assays for immunoglobulin and total protein can potentially distinguish primary hypogammaglobulinemia from protein loss. Exploring vaccine responses and assessing the lymphocyte profile may broadly indicate whether there is a humoral immune defect, a cellular defect, or a combination of both. Previous volumes in this tetralogy extensively covered immune defects and their gastrointestinal manifestations. This

This chapter is partially based on the chapter published in the book: Cellular Primary Immunodeficiencies, Springer, 2021, edited by Mario Milco D'Elios, Cosima Tatiana Baldari, Francesco Annunziato.

S. D'Elios
Department of Clinical and Experimental Medicine, University of Pisa, Pisa, Italy

M. Benagiano
Department of Experimental and Clinical Medicine, University of Florence, Florence, Italy

E. Asvestopoulou · M. M. D'Elios (✉) · C. Della Bella
Department of Molecular and Developmental Medicine, University of Siena, Siena, Italy
e-mail: delios@unisi.it

M. M. D'Elios (ed.), *Severe Combined Immunodeficiency*, Rare Diseases of the Immune System, https://doi.org/10.1007/978-3-031-78864-2_7

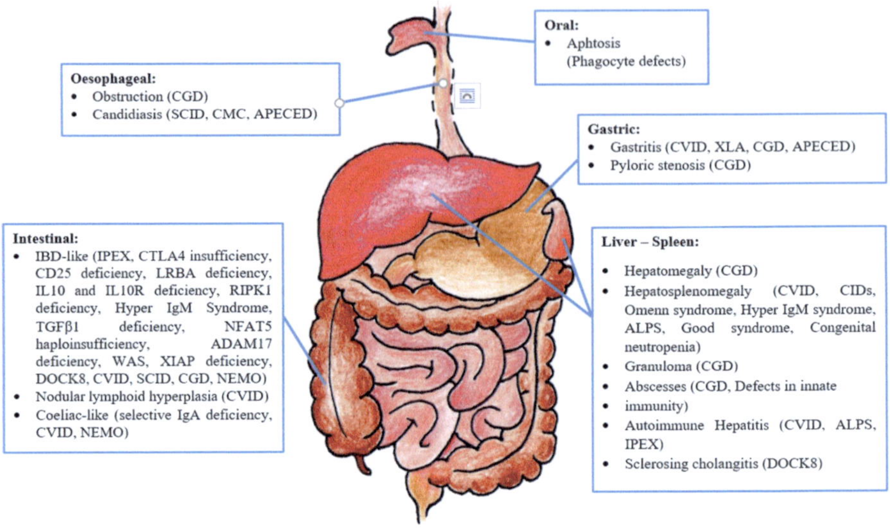

Fig. 7.1 Overview of primary immunodeficiencies affecting different parts of the gastrointestinal tract. Primary immunodeficiencies can affect any site of the gastrointestinal tract. Infections, inflammatory, autoimmune, and malignant manifestations may occur in PID patients

chapter will specifically delve into the gastrointestinal manifestations associated with primary cellular immunodeficiencies.

7.1 B and T Cell Defects

7.1.1 Severe Combined Immune Deficiency

Combined T and B immunodeficiencies, which impact both B cell and T cell functions, lead to gastrointestinal disorders that can be found in 90% of affected patients. If left untreated, these gastrointestinal issues can pose life-threatening risks [1, 2]. Diarrhea and malabsorption may arise from bacterial infections, with viral infections like rotavirus, cytomegalovirus, Epstein-Barr virus, adenovirus, or opportunistic infections like *P. aeruginosa* being more frequent culprits [3]. Notably, rotavirus vaccination has been shown to potentially lead to chronic infection in infants with severe combined immunodeficiency (SCID) [4]. Common gastrointestinal manifestations include candidiasis, affecting the oral, esophageal, perianal, and occasionally intestinal regions. Oral and esophageal candidiasis can contribute to failure to thrive by reducing oral intake in affected children [5]. Additionally, infections from *E. coli*, *Giardia*, *Cryptosporidium*, *Salmonella*, and *Shigella* have been documented [6]. Gastrointestinal symptoms may also occur due to graft-versus-host disease (GVHD) following bone marrow transplantation or blood transfusions.

Gastric and intestinal biopsies in severe combined immunodeficiency (SCID) patients reveal a hypocellular lamina propria devoid of lymphocytes or plasma cells. Notably, cytomegalovirus and adenovirus have been identified in gut biopsies of individuals with SCID. Infections may lead to villous atrophy. A GVHD-like process impacting the colon and small intestine has been documented not only in patients who underwent bone marrow transplantations or blood transfusions but also in pre-bone marrow transplantation biopsies [7, 8]. Infections and GVHD can extend their impact to the liver, where pathological conditions caused by adenovirus rotavirus and CMV hepatitis have been reported [9, 10]. Acute GVHD of the pancreas and occurrences of viral pancreatitis have also been observed [11].

7.1.2 DOCK8 Deficiency

Gastrointestinal viral infections, including those involving Epstein-Barr virus, rotavirus, herpes simplex virus, as well as hepatitis A, B, and C viruses, have been documented in DOCK8-deficient patients [12–15]. Additionally, hepatobiliary infection with *Cryptosporidium* has been described in these patients, posing challenges in terms of severity and treatment [16]. Parasitic infections documented in this peculiar DOCK8 immunodeficient context encompass *Entamoeba histolytica* and *Giardia lamblia* [13, 17, 18]. Sclerosing cholangitis, stemming from chronic infection, has been reported in DOCK8-deficient patients [17]. Furthermore, instances of eosinophilic esophagitis have been reported [19].

Complications in the intestinal tract may eventually result in failure to thrive and impaired growth [13].

Malabsorption, leading to failure to thrive, can stem not only from infections but also from allergic or autoimmune enteropathy. Chronic diarrhea induced by enteropathy can be so huge that it may mimic an IPEX-like disease [20].

7.1.3 NFKB Essential Modulator Deficiency (NEMO) Syndrome

X-linked recessive primary immune deficiency, resulting from a genetic mutation impacting the inhibitor of nuclear factor kappa-B kinase subunit gamma (IKBKG) gene, which encodes the NEMO protein, manifests as abnormal development of the immune system, affecting dendritic cells, phagocytes, and lymphocytes. Individuals with this pathological condition exhibit increased susceptiveness to bacterial and fungal infections. Gastrointestinal infections have been documented in over 20% of NEMO patients, with examples including severe adenoviral gastroenteritis [21].

A study conducted by Hanson et al. that characterized NEMO phenotypes revealed that 21% of patients exhibited inflammatory colitis. Nearly half of these individuals experienced refractory diarrhea and impaired growth [22]. Both the large and small intestine was involved in the inflammatory bowel disease observed in NEMO patients. Histologically, gut findings in these NEMO patients included acute inflammation, edema, superficial cryptitis, mucosal ulceration, and an abundance of neutrophils within the lamina propria [23].

7.1.4 Omenn Syndrome

An autosomal recessive form of severe combined immunodeficiency (SCID) is Omenn syndrome. This syndrome is characterized by impaired growth, lymphadenopathy, eosinophilia, hepatosplenomegaly, elevated serum IgE levels erythroderma, desquamation, alopecia, and chronic diarrhea. From a molecular point of view, Omenn syndrome can be ascribed to genetic defects in *RAG1*, *RAG2*, or *DCLRE1C/ARTEMIS*.

Patients affected by conditions such as *RAG1/RAG2* defects or *ARTEMIS* deficiency may manifest gastric and intestinal symptoms, including malabsorption, refractory diarrhea, enteric pathogens infections, as well as impaired growth. Enterocolitis resembling IBD has been reported in individuals with *RAG1*, *RAG2*, or *DCLRE1C/ARTEMIS* deficiencies [24, 25].

7.2 Congenital Defects of Phagocyte Number or Function

This section will primarily address defects in oxidative burst, which have been associated with distinct intestinal involvement. It is important to note that symptoms affecting the gastrointestinal tract can also be present in individuals with other deficiencies in phagocyte function and number. For instance, in a study involving 14 patients with glucose-6-phosphatase catalytic subunit 3 (G6PC3) deficiency, three patients developed Crohn's disease, while five experienced chronic diarrhea with steatorrhea [26].

7.2.1 Chronic Granulomatous Disease (CGD)

Gastrointestinal (GI) involvement is a prevalent and recurrent issue in chronic granulomatous disease (CGD), particularly in cases with X-linked inheritance [27]. CGD is a condition arising from defects in the subunits of the nicotinamide adenine dinucleotide phosphate (NADPH) oxidase enzyme complex within phagocytes. This enzyme complex plays a crucial role in generating superoxide anion radicals, essential for effectively killing catalase-positive organisms. Due to these defects, phagocytes in individuals with CGD are incapable of efficiently eliminating intracellular and some extracellular microorganisms [28]. As a result, patients with CGD experience recurrent, life-threatening bacterial and fungal infections shortly after birth. These infections can impact various areas, including the skin, gastrointestinal and respiratory tracts, as well as other organs where a high number of phagocytes are present, such as the liver [29].

The most commonly encountered pathogens in chronic granulomatous disease (CGD) include *Staphylococcus aureus*, *Burkholderia cepacia*, *Serratia marcescens*,

Aspergillus species, *Chromobacterium violaceum*, and *Nocardia* species [30]. Despite improvements in the average survival age of CGD patients, infections remain a significant contributor to mortality. In a study conducted by Yu et al., serum levels of antibodies specific to gastrointestinal pathogens were measured in CGD patients, revealing elevated levels of these antibodies. However, these levels did not exhibit a correlation with the presence or absence of intestinal inflammation, and thus, they did not provide an explanation for the etiopathogenesis of intestinal manifestations [31].

Approximately 70% of chronic granulomatous disease (CGD) patients exhibit gastrointestinal symptoms such as non-infectious diarrhea, oral aphthosis, anal fistulas, vomiting, anorexia, and abdominal pain [32, 33]. Gastrointestinal involvement in CGD can resemble other inflammatory bowel diseases, manifesting as Crohn-like disease, protein-losing enteropathy, or noncaseating granulomatous colitis. Granulomata can affect the entire gastrointestinal tract, leading to symptoms like dysphagia, dysmotility, or obstruction [34].

In a study involving 87 chronic granulomatous disease (CGD) patients with gastrointestinal symptoms who underwent endoscopy, 95% of those with such symptoms displayed pathological histological findings. These findings included the frequent presence of micrognanulomas, pigmented macrophages, and eosinophils in both acute and chronic inflammation, irrespective of the presence of neutrophils. The colon was the most commonly affected segment of the gastrointestinal tract. Some biopsies from the duodenum and ileum showed villi shortening. Establishing a correlation between inflammatory infiltrates and a triggering infection was almost never feasible [35]. In a retrospective study of 20 CGD patients with inflammatory gastrointestinal manifestations, 55% reported nonspecific diarrhea, with severe endoscopic appearances not consistently aligning with the severity of symptoms. The colon was extensively involved in 44% of the patients, and characteristic features such as epithelioid granulomas, pigmented macrophages, and increased eosinophils were present in 78% of patients [36].

The treatment of gastrointestinal involvement in chronic granulomatous disease (CGD) often involves antibiotics or other anti-infective agents, steroids, and various immunomodulatory or immunosuppressive therapies. However, the benefits of these interventions must be carefully weighed against the risk of infectious complications. In some cases, surgery may be considered. For severely affected patients, hematopoietic stem cell transplantation is an option. The choice of treatment strategy depends on the specific manifestations and severity of gastrointestinal symptoms in each individual case.

Hepatic involvement is a common occurrence in chronic granulomatous disease (CGD). Liver abscesses represent a frequent complication, with *S. aureus* and *Pseudomonas aeruginosa* often identified as the causative pathogens. Approximately 27% of CGD patients have reported abscesses with *S. aureus* [37]. Additionally, drug-induced hepatotoxicity is a frequent concern. Other hepatic manifestations include nodular regenerative hyperplasia and hepatosplenomegaly [38]. The microvascular structures of the liver may sustain vascular injuries from repeated systemic and hepatic infections, potentially leading to noncirrhotic portal hypertension, which is associated with a high mortality rate [39].

7.2.2 Leukocyte Adhesion Deficiency Type 1

Leukocyte adhesion deficiency type 1 (LAD-1) is an autosomal recessive primary immunodeficiency resulting from mutations in the integrin β2 gene (ITGB2), which encodes the common β subunit of the β2 integrin family, also known as CD18. The dysfunction of integrins leads to impaired leukocyte adhesion to the vascular wall, hindering the migration of polymorphonuclear (PMN) cells to tissue sites and preventing the formation of pus [40]. This condition is accompanied by neutrophilia. Patients with LAD-1 typically exhibit omphalitis during the newborn period, non-purulent skin and soft tissue infections, perirectal abscesses, periodontitis, and defective wound healing [41, 42]. The most common pathogens associated with LAD-1 include *Staphylococcus aureus*, *Pseudomonas aeruginosa*, *Klebsiella* species, and fungal infections may also occur [43].

In addition to the previously mentioned symptoms, other gastrointestinal manifestations of leukocyte adhesion deficiency type 1 (LAD-1) include diarrhea and hepatosplenomegaly. Moreover, there have been reports of chronic ileocolitis that resembles idiopathic inflammatory bowel disease (IBD), characterized by inflammation and ulceration affecting the colon and the terminal ileum [44, 45]. It is worth noting that cord blood transplantation has been observed to lead to remission of the IBD-like disease in some cases [46].

7.3 Diseases of Immune Dysregulation

The gastrointestinal system is often regarded as the largest lymphoid organ in the body, with its lumen densely populated by vast numbers of microorganisms that regularly come into contact with resident immune cells. Additionally, the presence of food antigens poses a continuous challenge. Consequently, tight regulation is essential to maintain homeostasis, and the functions of the barrier, as well as the preservation of tolerance, are of utmost importance. In immune dysregulation syndromes, these regulatory mechanisms fail, leading to the association of many of these syndromes with enteropathy and gastrointestinal inflammation. In this context, we present several characteristic examples, though it is important to note that this list is by no means exhaustive, as patients with almost any immunodysregulatory disease may develop gastrointestinal manifestations.

7.3.1 Regulatory T Cell Defects

7.3.1.1 IPEX Syndrome

The immune dysregulation polyendocrinopathy X-linked (IPEX) syndrome arises from mutations in the transcription factor FOXP3, leading to the dysfunction of regulatory T cells and subsequent immune dysregulation and susceptibility to autoimmunity [47]. IPEX syndrome is characterized by severe enteropathy, often intractable, and early-onset polyendocrinopathy, frequently involving type 1 diabetes.

Enteropathy manifests as refractory secretory, i.e., watery, but sometimes also bloody diarrhea in the first months of life and often does not respond to enteric rest [48]. Consequently, patients frequently experience failure to thrive and malnutrition, necessitating total parenteral nutrition.

As a result of the loss of oral tolerance, patients with IPEX syndrome may exhibit severe food allergies, and IgE levels can be elevated [49]. Autoantibodies such as anti-enterocyte, anti-harmonin, or anti-villin are often detectable in individuals with enteropathy [50, 51].

Enteropathy may contribute to protein loss, including hypogammaglobulinemia. Additionally, severe enteropathy may facilitate the translocation of bacteria from the gut, potentially leading to infectious complications.

Histopathological observations often reveal partial or total villous atrophy with mucosal erosion and ulcerations, potentially progressing to the destruction of the small bowel mucosa in IPEX syndrome. A characteristic finding is the presence of lymphocytic infiltrates in the lamina propria and submucosa, which may extend to other organs [50, 52]. Colon involvement is also possible. Treatment typically involves total parenteral nutrition and immunosuppressive agents such as cyclosporin A, tacrolimus, sirolimus, and corticosteroids. However, it is important to note that immunosuppression may increase the risk of opportunistic infections [53, 54]. Hematopoietic stem cell transplantation represents a curative approach and has been shown to lead to gut immune reconstitution [55, 56].

7.3.1.2 CD25 Deficiency

CD25 deficiency is a rare regulatory T cell defect that results in an IPEX-like syndrome [57]. Patients with this condition often exhibit severe early-onset autoimmune enteropathy, characterized by chronic diarrhea similar to that seen in IPEX. Protein loss may also accompany these gastrointestinal symptoms. Histopathological findings in CD25 deficiency resemble those observed in IPEX, with prominent villous atrophy [58]. Notably, individuals with CD25 deficiency tend to have a higher susceptibility to various infections, including viral, bacterial, and fungal infections, often of opportunistic nature. This heightened vulnerability can complicate the management of the condition with immunosuppressive treatment [57, 59]. Hematopoietic stem cell transplantation is considered a curative approach for CD25 deficiency [58].

7.3.1.3 CTLA4 Insufficiency

CTLA4 insufficiency is likely the most prevalent regulatory T cell defect and is frequently linked to gastrointestinal complications. A study by Schwab et al. revealed that 59% of patients with CTLA4 insufficiency experienced gastrointestinal involvement although the severity varied among individuals [60]. Diarrhea is a prevalent symptom, and some patients received a concurrent diagnosis of Crohn's disease [61]. Additionally, cases of atrophic gastritis have been reported. Histopathological observations include ulcerative lesions, deep T cell infiltrates, and inflammatory alterations in the submucosa.

Treatment with CTLA4 fusion proteins, such as abatacept and belatacept, has shown promise in improving clinical symptoms, including enteropathy, in individuals with CTLA4 insufficiency.

7.3.1.4 LRBA Deficiency

For a comprehensive understanding of LRBA deficiency, detailed information can be found in the second book of the series titled *Humoral Primary Immunodeficiencies* [62].

7.3.2 Immune Dysregulation with Colitis

7.3.2.1 IL10 and IL10R Deficiency

IL10 plays a crucial role as an immunoregulatory cytokine, being produced by various cell types, including regulatory T cells, monocytes, macrophages, B cells, and epithelial cells. Loss-of-function mutations in IL10, IL10RA, or IL10RB can result in very early-onset inflammatory bowel disease, typically emerging within the first year of life [63, 64]. Affected individuals exhibit severe and challenging-to-treat enterocolitis, often accompanied by perianal disease, fistula formation, and failure to thrive. Besides gastrointestinal symptoms, patients may experience extraintestinal manifestations like folliculitis, recurrent respiratory disease, and arthritis [65]. Immunological assessments typically reveal subtle abnormalities, such as alterations in the CD4/CD8 T cell ratio and variable immunoglobulin levels.

Histopathological observations in IL10-related inflammatory bowel disease may encompass ulcerations, pseudopolyps, granulation, inflammatory infiltrates, and abscesses.

The disease often proves refractory to conventional immunosuppressive treatment, necessitating surgical interventions. Hematopoietic stem cell transplantation stands as a curative approach [65, 66].

7.3.2.2 RIPK1 Deficiency

RIPK1 deficiency results in a primary immunodeficiency characterized by immune dysregulation and intestinal inflammation. Depending on the genetic mutation, patients may either present with a combined immunodeficiency phenotype, including diarrhea, or with a predominantly early-onset IBD phenotype [67]. Other extraintestinal manifestations encompass progressive polyarthritis [68]. Patients exhibit lymphopenia with impaired B and T cell differentiation and an increased susceptibility to recurrent viral, bacterial, and fungal infections. Limited data are available, but histologic features of RIPK1 deficiency include chronic inflammation with erosions, increased apoptotic bodies within the cryptic bases, and depletion of lamina propria plasma cells [67]. Hematopoietic stem cell transplantation has shown effectiveness in addressing immunodeficiency, enteropathy, and arthritis [68].

7.3.2.3 NFAT5 Haploinsufficiency

Boland et al. reported a patient with a heterozygous mutation in NFAT5 who developed an IBD-like autoimmune enteropathy beginning at the age of 7 years.

Histopathological observations comprised intraepithelial lymphocytosis, abundant apoptotic enterocytes, and an absence of goblet cells, with positive anti-goblet cell antibodies. The patient also experienced extraintestinal manifestations such as eczema and recurrent respiratory tract infections [69].

7.3.2.4 TGFB1 Deficiency

In 2018, Kotlarz et al. reported three patients from two families with TGFB1 deficiency, showcasing severe, very early-onset inflammatory bowel disease and encephalopathy, which encompassed epilepsy, brain atrophy, and global developmental delay [70]. Two of the three patients also suffered from recurrent infections. Histological examinations revealed inflammatory infiltrates in the epithelium with mucosal ulceration and crypt abscesses. Tragically, two of the three patients underwent rapid neurological deterioration and ultimately succumbed to infectious complications at the ages of 25 and 39 months [70].

7.3.2.5 ADAM17 Deficiency

ADAM17, also known as TNF-α-converting enzyme (TACE), is a metalloproteinase or sheddase crucial for shedding TNF-α from the cell surface. Deletion of *ADAM17* has been associated with inflammatory skin and bowel disease characterized by early-onset chronic diarrhea and failure to thrive [71]. The diarrhea is malabsorptive and bloody, accompanied by an inflammatory skin condition featuring psoriasiform erythroderma and generalized pustular rashes. PBMCs from affected patients demonstrated impaired TNF-α production. Presently, only two patients from a single kindred have been reported with this condition.

7.3.3 Immune Dysregulation with Lymphoproliferative Defects

7.3.3.1 XIAP Deficiency

XIAP deficiency, or X-linked lymphoproliferative syndrome type 2 (XLP2), is a clinically diverse immune dysregulation syndrome that can manifest as EBV-triggered lymphoproliferative disease, splenomegaly, hemophagocytic lymphohistiocytosis (HLH), and a Crohn-like enteropathy. Depending on the cohort, 0–29% of patients may experience colitis/enteropathy [72–74]. Atypical presentations of (very) early-onset inflammatory bowel disease (IBD) are common in XIAP deficiency [75, 76]. In a cohort described by Aguilar et al., IBD was the primary or most severe clinical finding in half of the XIAP-deficient patients [72]. Even female carriers with skewed X-inactivation toward the mutated allele may develop an IBD phenotype [72, 77]. Patients initially presenting with IBD may subsequently develop HLH. IBD in XIAP deficiency is often severe, accompanied by abscess formation, perineal fistulae, and is challenging to treat. The distribution of symptoms often mimics Crohn's disease. Histopathological findings include crypt abscesses, infiltrates, and epithelioid granulomas. Treatment is frequently refractory to immunosuppressive medication, necessitating aggressive interventions such as surgery.

Hematopoietic stem cell transplantation may lead to resolution of IBD and could be considered, especially in young patients, to prevent HLH [76, 78].

7.4 Defined Syndromes with Immunodeficiency and Gastrointestinal Involvement

7.4.1 Wiskott-Aldrich Syndrome

Wiskott-Aldrich syndrome (WAS) is a rare X-linked immune deficiency characterized by eczema, thrombocytopenia, and recurrent sinopulmonary infections, attributed to disruptions in the cytoskeletal integrity [79]. This syndrome is associated with a heightened risk of autoimmunity, including cytopenias, vasculitis, arthritis, and inflammatory bowel disease (IBD). In WAS, inflammatory bowel disease often manifests with symptoms like bloody diarrhea and malabsorption [80]. It can present as either ulcerative colitis or Crohn's disease and is observed in approximately 10% of patients [81, 82]. Endoscopic and histopathological findings may include a cobblestone appearance, inflammatory pseudopolyps, cryptitis, and crypt abscesses although limited data on histopathology exist due to the elevated risk of bleeding complications during procedures [82, 83]. Laboratory findings may reveal eosinophilia, elevated IgE levels, and specific IgE to food allergens [84, 85]. It is noteworthy that individuals with mutations in WAS may also present with a (very) early-onset IBD phenotype even in the absence of the classic triad of thrombocytopenia, eczema, and susceptibility to infections [86].

Treatment options for Wiskott-Aldrich syndrome (WAS)-associated inflammatory bowel disease (IBD) include immunosuppressive approaches like steroids or cyclosporin. For severe cases, more advanced interventions such as gene therapy and hematopoietic stem cell transplantation may be considered. The choice of treatment depends on the severity of the symptoms and the specific clinical profile of the individual patient [80, 87, 88].

7.4.2 DiGeorge Syndrome

DiGeorge syndrome is characterized by thymic aplasia, leading to impaired T lymphocyte maturation, while B cells are typically unaffected [89]. The syndrome is associated with an increased frequency of autoimmune diseases, including autoimmune enteropathy and celiac disease [90]. A study evaluating 26 patients with DiGeorge syndrome found gastrointestinal (GI) involvement in 58% of patients. Symptoms may include abdominal pain, vomiting, gastroesophageal reflux, chronic constipation, and abnormal intestinal permeability [91]. Complete DiGeorge syndrome, where patients lack a thymus, may present shortly after birth with recurrent severe infections, chronic diarrhea, and failure to thrive. This form of the disease is fatal unless a thymus or bone marrow transplant is performed [92]. Additionally,

22q11 deletion syndromes, which encompass DiGeorge syndrome, may involve structural defects in the laryngotracheoesophageal and gastrointestinal systems. These defects may include cleft lip/palate, velopharyngeal incompetence leading to dysphagia and feeding difficulties, esophageal atresia, mal- or nonrotation, and Hirschsprung disease [93–96].

7.4.3 Chronic Mucocutaneous Candidiasis and APECED Syndrome

Disorders marked by compromised T cell proliferation and cytokine production in response to *Candida albicans* antigens characterize these syndromes. Candida esophagitis, stemming from these immunodeficiencies, can lead to diminished oral intake and failure to thrive.

Autoimmune polyendocrinopathy-candidiasis-ectodermal dystrophy (APECED) syndrome, resulting from mutations in the AIRE gene, includes autoimmune gastritis and pancreatic insufficiency among its manifestations, contributing to weight loss as gastrointestinal symptoms [97, 98].

7.5 Conclusions

Patients with primary immunodeficiencies (PIDs) often exhibit gastrointestinal (GI) symptoms that can significantly impact their health, and in some cases, lead to increased mortality. The GI manifestations of PIDs may resemble those of common gastrointestinal diseases, posing challenges in diagnosis, particularly when GI symptoms precede other signs of PID. Uncommonly severe or persistent infections that do not respond to typical treatments, along with the identification of unusual pathogens, may raise suspicion of an underlying immune system defect. Early recognition and diagnosis of PID are crucial for appropriate management and improved outcomes.

Indeed, inflammatory bowel disease (IBD)-like disease is a frequent manifestation of cellular immunodeficiencies, and its early onset should raise suspicion of an underlying immune defect. This is particularly relevant in regions where consanguineous marriages are common.

Flow cytometric analysis and phagocytic respiratory burst tests can serve as initial screening tools for the most common cellular immunodeficiencies associated with the clinical presentation. Additionally, T cell receptor excision circle (TREC) analysis is valuable for screening severe combined immunodeficiency (SCID). However, as genetic analysis has become more accessible, it is increasingly considered as a comprehensive diagnostic approach. In cases of very early-onset inflammatory bowel disease (IBD), genetic analysis can aid in identifying underlying genetic defects. This information not only helps anticipate potential future disease manifestations but also informs treatment decisions, particularly for severely affected patients.

References

1. Lai Ping So A, Mayer L (1997) Gastrointestinal manifestations of primary immunodeficiency disorders. Semin Gastrointest Dis 8(1):22–32
2. Rosen FS (1986) Defects in cell-mediated immunity. Clin Immunol Immunopathol 41(1):1–7
3. Jarvis WR, Middleton PJ, Gelfand EW (1983) Significance of viral infections in severe combined immunodeficiency disease. Pediatr Infect Dis 2(3):187–192
4. Bakare N, Menschik D, Tiernan R, Hua W, Martin D (2010) Severe combined immunodeficiency (SCID) and rotavirus vaccination: reports to the Vaccine Adverse Events Reporting System (VAERS). Vaccine 28(40):6609–6612
5. Patil S, Rao RS, Majumdar B, Anil S (2015) Clinical appearance of oral candida infection and therapeutic strategies. Front Microbiol 6:1391
6. Stephan JL, Vlekova V, Le Deist F, Blanche S, Donadieu J, De Saint-Basile G et al (1993) Severe combined immunodeficiency: a retrospective single-center study of clinical presentation and outcome in 117 patients. J Pediatr 123(4):564–572
7. Snover DC, Filipovich AH, Ramsay NK, Weisdorf SA, Kersey JH (1985) Graft-versus-host-disease-like histopathological findings in pre-bone-marrow transplantation biopsies of patients with severe T cell deficiency. Transplantation 39(1):95–97
8. Lee EY, Clouse RE, Aliperti G, DeSchryver-Kecskemeti K (1991) Small intestinal lesion resembling graft-vs-host disease. A case report in immunodeficiency and review of the literature. Arch Pathol Lab Med 115(5):529–532
9. Washington K, Gossage DL, Gottfried MR (1993) Pathology of the liver in severe combined immunodeficiency and DiGeorge syndrome. Pediatr Pathol 13(4):485–504
10. Gilger MA, Matson DO, Conner ME, Rosenblatt HM, Finegold MJ, Estes MK (1992) Extraintestinal rotavirus infections in children with immunodeficiency. J Pediatr 120(6):912–917
11. Washington K, Gossage DL, Gottfried MR (1994) Pathology of the pancreas in severe combined immunodeficiency and DiGeorge syndrome: acute graft-versus-host disease and unusual viral infections. Hum Pathol 25(9):908–914
12. Sanal O, Jing H, Ozgur T, Ayvaz D, Strauss-Albee DM, Ersoy-Evans S et al (2012) Additional diverse findings expand the clinical presentation of DOCK8 deficiency. J Clin Immunol 32(4):698–708
13. Engelhardt KR, Gertz ME, Keles S, Schäffer AA, Sigmund EC, Glocker C et al (2015) The extended clinical phenotype of 64 patients with dedicator of cytokinesis 8 deficiency. J Allergy Clin Immunol 136(2):402–412
14. Alsum Z, Hawwari A, Alsmadi O, Al-Hissi S, Borrero E, Abu-Staiteh A et al (2013) Clinical, immunological and molecular characterization of DOCK8 and DOCK8-like deficient patients: single center experience of twenty-five patients. J Clin Immunol 33(1):55–67
15. Betts K, Abusleme L, Freeman AF, Sarmadi M, Fahle G, Pittaluga S et al (2015) A 17-year old patient with DOCK8 deficiency, severe oral HSV-1 and aggressive periodontitis—a case of virally induced periodontitis? J Clin Virol 63:46–50
16. Al-Herz W, Ragupathy R, Massaad MJ, Al-Attiyah R, Nanda A, Engelhardt KR et al (2012) Clinical, immunologic and genetic profiles of DOCK8-deficient patients in Kuwait. Clin Immunol 143(3):266–272
17. Shah T, Cale C, Hadzic N, Jones A (2014) Dedicator of cytokinesis 8 deficiency: a predisposition to sclerosing cholangitis. Clin Immunol 155(1):71–73
18. Al-Herz W, Chu JI, van der Spek J, Raghupathy R, Massaad MJ, Keles S et al (2016) Hematopoietic stem cell transplantation outcomes for 11 patients with dedicator of cytokinesis 8 deficiency. J Allergy Clin Immunol 138(3):852–859.e3
19. Biggs CM, Keles S, Chatila TA (2017) DOCK8 deficiency: insights into pathophysiology, clinical features and management. Clin Immunol 181:75–82
20. Alroqi FJ, Charbonnier LM, Keles S, Ghandour F, Mouawad P, Sabouneh R et al (2017) DOCK8 deficiency presenting as an IPEX-like disorder. J Clin Immunol 37(8):811–819

21. Picard C, Casanova JL, Puel A (2011) Infectious diseases in patients with IRAK-4, MyD88, NEMO, or IκBα deficiency. Clin Microbiol Rev 24(3):490–497
22. Hanson EP, Monaco-Shawver L, Solt LA, Madge LA, Banerjee PP, May MJ et al (2008) Hypomorphic nuclear factor-kappaB essential modulator mutation database and reconstitution system identifies phenotypic and immunologic diversity. J Allergy Clin Immunol 122(6):1169–1177.e16
23. Cheng LE, Kanwar B, Tcheurekdjian H, Grenert JP, Muskat M, Heyman MB et al (2009) Persistent systemic inflammation and atypical enterocolitis in patients with NEMO syndrome. Clin Immunol 132(1):124–131
24. Hönig M, Schwarz K (2006) Omenn syndrome: a lack of tolerance on the background of deficient lymphocyte development and maturation. Curr Opin Rheumatol 18(4):383–388
25. Puzenat E, Rohrlich P, Thierry P, Girardin P, Taghian M, Ouachee M et al (2007) Omenn syndrome: a rare case of neonatal erythroderma. Eur J Dermatol 17(2):137–139
26. Desplantes C, Fremond ML, Beaupain B, Harousseau JL, Buzyn A, Pellier I et al (2014) Clinical spectrum and long-term follow-up of 14 cases with G6PC3 mutations from the French Severe Congenital Neutropenia Registry. Orphanet J Rare Dis 9:183
27. Marciano BE, Rosenzweig SD, Kleiner DE, Anderson VL, Darnell DN, Anaya-O'Brien S et al (2004) Gastrointestinal involvement in chronic granulomatous disease. Pediatrics 114(2):462–468
28. Arnold DE, Heimall JR (2017) A review of chronic granulomatous disease. Adv Ther 34(12):2543–2557
29. Marciano BE, Spalding C, Fitzgerald A, Mann D, Brown T, Osgood S et al (2015) Common severe infections in chronic granulomatous disease. Clin Infect Dis 60(8):1176–1183
30. McCabe RP (2002) Gastrointestinal manifestations of non-AIDS immunodeficiency. Curr Treat Opt Gastroenterol 5(1):17–25
31. Yu JE, De Ravin SS, Uzel G, Landers C, Targan S, Malech HL et al (2011) High levels of Crohn's disease-associated anti-microbial antibodies are present and independent of colitis in chronic granulomatous disease. Clin Immunol 138(1):14–22
32. Rieber N, Hector A, Kuijpers T, Roos D, Hartl D (2012) Current concepts of hyperinflammation in chronic granulomatous disease. Clin Dev Immunol 2012:252460
33. van den Berg JM, van Koppen E, Ahlin A, Belohradsky BH, Bernatowska E, Corbeel L et al (2009) Chronic granulomatous disease: the European experience. PLoS One 4(4):e5234
34. Magnani A, Brosselin P, Beauté J, de Vergnes N, Mouy R, Debré M et al (2014) Inflammatory manifestations in a single-center cohort of patients with chronic granulomatous disease. J Allergy Clin Immunol 134(3):655–662.e8
35. Alimchandani M, Lai JP, Aung PP, Khangura S, Kamal N, Gallin JI et al (2013) Gastrointestinal histopathology in chronic granulomatous disease: a study of 87 patients. Am J Surg Pathol 37(9):1365–1372
36. Angelino G, De Angelis P, Faraci S, Rea F, Romeo EF, Torroni F et al (2017) Inflammatory bowel disease in chronic granulomatous disease: an emerging problem over a twenty years' experience. Pediatr Allergy Immunol 28(8):801–809
37. Winkelstein JA, Marino MC, Johnston RB, Boyle J, Curnutte J, Gallin JI et al (2000) Chronic granulomatous disease. Report on a national registry of 368 patients. Medicine (Baltimore) 79(3):155–169
38. Hussain N, Feld JJ, Kleiner DE, Hoofnagle JH, Garcia-Eulate R, Ahlawat S et al (2007) Hepatic abnormalities in patients with chronic granulomatous disease. Hepatology 45(3):675–683
39. Feld JJ, Hussain N, Wright EC, Kleiner DE, Hoofnagle JH, Ahlawat S et al (2008) Hepatic involvement and portal hypertension predict mortality in chronic granulomatous disease. Gastroenterology 134(7):1917–1926
40. Etzioni A (2009) Genetic etiologies of leukocyte adhesion defects. Curr Opin Immunol 21(5):481–486
41. Levy-Mendelovich S, Rechavi E, Abuzaitoun O, Vernitsky H, Simon AJ, Lev A et al (2016) Highlighting the problematic reliance on CD18 for diagnosing leukocyte adhesion deficiency type 1. Immunol Res 64(2):476–482

42. Roberts MW, Atkinson JC (1990) Oral manifestations associated with leukocyte adhesion deficiency: a five-year case study. Pediatr Dent 12(2):107–111
43. Wolach B, Gavrieli R, Wolach O, Stauber T, Abuzaitoun O, Kuperman A et al (2019) Leucocyte adhesion deficiency—a multicentre national experience. Eur J Clin Investig 49(2):e13047
44. D'Agata ID, Paradis K, Chad Z, Bonny Y, Seidman E (1996) Leucocyte adhesion deficiency presenting as a chronic ileocolitis. Gut 39(4):605–608
45. Uzel G, Kleiner DE, Kuhns DB, Holland SM (2001) Dysfunctional LAD-1 neutrophils and colitis. Gastroenterology 121(4):958–964
46. Jain S, Gozdziak P, Morgan A, Burt RK (2013) Remission of Crohn's disease after cord blood transplantation for leukocyte adhesion deficiency type 1. Bone Marrow Transplant 48(7):1006–1007
47. Chatila TA, Blaeser F, Ho N, Lederman HM, Voulgaropoulos C, Helms C et al (2000) JM2, encoding a fork head-related protein, is mutated in X-linked autoimmunity-allergic disregulation syndrome. J Clin Invest 106(12):R75–R81
48. Wildin RS, Smyk-Pearson S, Filipovich AH (2002) Clinical and molecular features of the immunodysregulation, polyendocrinopathy, enteropathy, X linked (IPEX) syndrome. J Med Genet 39(8):537–545
49. Torgerson TR, Linane A, Moes N, Anover S, Mateo V, Rieux-Laucat F et al (2007) Severe food allergy as a variant of IPEX syndrome caused by a deletion in a noncoding region of the FOXP3 gene. Gastroenterology 132(5):1705–1717
50. Patey-Mariaud de Serre N, Canioni D, Ganousse S, Rieux-Laucat F, Goulet O, Ruemmele F et al (2009) Digestive histopathological presentation of IPEX syndrome. Mod Pathol 22(1):95–102
51. Barzaghi F, Amaya Hernandez LC, Neven B, Ricci S, Kucuk ZY, Bleesing JJ et al (2018) Long-term follow-up of IPEX syndrome patients after different therapeutic strategies: an international multicenter retrospective study. J Allergy Clin Immunol 141(3):1036–1049.e5
52. Bennett CL, Ochs HD (2001) IPEX is a unique X-linked syndrome characterized by immune dysfunction, polyendocrinopathy, enteropathy, and a variety of autoimmune phenomena. Curr Opin Pediatr 13(6):533–538
53. Yong PL, Russo P, Sullivan KE (2008) Use of sirolimus in IPEX and IPEX-like children. J Clin Immunol 28(5):581–587
54. Kobayashi I, Kawamura N, Okano M (2001) A long-term survivor with the immune dysregulation, polyendocrinopathy, enteropathy, X-linked syndrome. N Engl J Med 345(13):999–1000
55. Gambineri E, Ciullini Mannurita S, Robertson H, Vignoli M, Haugk B, Lionetti P et al (2015) Gut immune reconstitution in immune dysregulation, polyendocrinopathy, enteropathy, X-linked syndrome after hematopoietic stem cell transplantation. J Allergy Clin Immunol 135(1):260–262
56. Rao A, Kamani N, Filipovich A, Lee SM, Davies SM, Dalal J et al (2007) Successful bone marrow transplantation for IPEX syndrome after reduced-intensity conditioning. Blood 109(1):383–385
57. Caudy AA, Reddy ST, Chatila T, Atkinson JP, Verbsky JW (2007) CD25 deficiency causes an immune dysregulation, polyendocrinopathy, enteropathy, X-linked-like syndrome, and defective IL-10 expression from CD4 lymphocytes. J Allergy Clin Immunol 119(2):482–487
58. Vignoli M, Ciullini Mannurita S, Fioravanti A, Tumino M, Grassi A, Guariso G et al (2019) CD25 deficiency: a new conformational mutation prevents the receptor expression on cell surface. Clin Immunol 201:15–19
59. Sharfe N, Dadi HK, Shahar M, Roifman CM (1997) Human immune disorder arising from mutation of the alpha chain of the interleukin-2 receptor. Proc Natl Acad Sci USA 94(7):3168–3171
60. Schwab C, Gabrysch A, Olbrich P, Patiño V, Warnatz K, Wolff D et al (2018) Phenotype, penetrance, and treatment of 133 cytotoxic T-lymphocyte antigen 4-insufficient subjects. J Allergy Clin Immunol 142(6):1932–1946
61. Schubert D, Bode C, Kenefeck R, Hou TZ, Wing JB, Kennedy A et al (2014) Autosomal dominant immune dysregulation syndrome in humans with CTLA4 mutations. Nat Med 20(12):1410–1416

62. D'Elios MM, Rizzi M (2019) Humoral primary immunodeficiencies. Springer, Cham
63. Glocker EO, Kotlarz D, Boztug K, Gertz EM, Schaffer AA, Noyan F et al (2009) Inflammatory bowel disease and mutations affecting the interleukin-10 receptor. N Engl J Med 361(21):2033–2045
64. Glocker EO, Frede N, Perro M, Sebire N, Elawad M, Shah N et al (2010) Infant colitis—it's in the genes. Lancet 376(9748):1272
65. Engelhardt KR, Shah N, Faizura-Yeop I, Kocacik Uygun DF, Frede N, Muise AM et al (2013) Clinical outcome in IL-10- and IL-10 receptor-deficient patients with or without hematopoietic stem cell transplantation. J Allergy Clin Immunol 131(3):825–830
66. Kotlarz D, Beier R, Murugan D, Diestelhorst J, Jensen O, Boztug K et al (2012) Loss of interleukin-10 signaling and infantile inflammatory bowel disease: implications for diagnosis and therapy. Gastroenterology 143(2):347–355
67. Li Y, Führer M, Bahrami E, Socha P, Klaudel-Dreszler M, Bouzidi A et al (2019) Human RIPK1 deficiency causes combined immunodeficiency and inflammatory bowel diseases. Proc Natl Acad Sci USA 116(3):970–975
68. Cuchet-Lourenço D, Eletto D, Wu C, Plagnol V, Papapietro O, Curtis J et al (2018) Biallelic. Science 361(6404):810–813
69. Boland BS, Widjaja CE, Banno A, Zhang B, Kim SH, Stoven S et al (2015) Immunodeficiency and autoimmune enterocolopathy linked to NFAT5 haploinsufficiency. J Immunol 194(6):2551–2560
70. Kotlarz D, Marquardt B, Barøy T, Lee WS, Konnikova L, Hollizeck S et al (2018) Human TGF-β1 deficiency causes severe inflammatory bowel disease and encephalopathy. Nat Genet 50(3):344–348
71. Blaydon DC, Biancheri P, Di WL, Plagnol V, Cabral RM, Brooke MA et al (2011) Inflammatory skin and bowel disease linked to ADAM17 deletion. N Engl J Med 365(16):1502–1508
72. Aguilar C, Lenoir C, Lambert N, Bègue B, Brousse N, Canioni D et al (2014) Characterization of Crohn disease in X-linked inhibitor of apoptosis-deficient male patients and female symptomatic carriers. J Allergy Clin Immunol 134(5):1131–1141.e9
73. Marsh RA, Madden L, Kitchen BJ, Mody R, McClimon B, Jordan MB et al (2010) XIAP deficiency: a unique primary immunodeficiency best classified as X-linked familial hemophagocytic lymphohistiocytosis and not as X-linked lymphoproliferative disease. Blood 116(7):1079–1082
74. Yang X, Kanegane H, Nishida N, Imamura T, Hamamoto K, Miyashita R et al (2012) Clinical and genetic characteristics of XIAP deficiency in Japan. J Clin Immunol 32(3):411–420
75. Worthey EA, Mayer AN, Syverson GD, Helbling D, Bonacci BB, Decker B et al (2011) Making a definitive diagnosis: successful clinical application of whole exome sequencing in a child with intractable inflammatory bowel disease. Genet Med 13(3):255–262
76. Girardelli M, Arrigo S, Barabino A, Loganes C, Morreale G, Crovella S et al (2015) The diagnostic challenge of very early-onset enterocolitis in an infant with XIAP deficiency. BMC Pediatr 15:208
77. Dziadzio M, Ammann S, Canning C, Boyle F, Hassan A, Cale C et al (2015) Symptomatic males and female carriers in a large Caucasian kindred with XIAP deficiency. J Clin Immunol 35(5):439–444
78. Tsuma Y, Imamura T, Ichise E, Sakamoto K, Ouchi K, Osone S et al (2015) Successful treatment of idiopathic colitis related to XIAP deficiency with allo-HSCT using reduced-intensity conditioning. Pediatr Transplant 19(1):E25–E28
79. Candotti F (2018) Clinical manifestations and pathophysiological mechanisms of the Wiskott-Aldrich syndrome. J Clin Immunol 38(1):13–27
80. Dupuis-Girod S, Medioni J, Haddad E, Quartier P, Cavazzana-Calvo M, Le Deist F et al (2003) Autoimmunity in Wiskott-Aldrich syndrome: risk factors, clinical features, and outcome in a single-center cohort of 55 patients. Pediatrics 111(5 Pt 1):e622–e627
81. Folwaczny C, Ruelfs C, Walther J, König A, Emmerich B (2002) Ulcerative colitis in a patient with Wiskott-Aldrich syndrome. Endoscopy 34(10):840–841

82. Hsieh KH, Chang MH, Lee CY, Wang CY (1988) Wiskott-Aldrich syndrome and inflammatory bowel disease. Ann Allergy 60(5):429–431
83. Esmaeilzadeh H, Bordbar MR, Dastsooz H, Silawi M, Fard MAF, Adib A et al (2018) A novel splice site mutation in WAS gene in patient with Wiskott-Aldrich syndrome and chronic colitis: a case report. BMC Med Genet 19(1):123
84. Root AW, Speicher CE (1963) The triad of thrombocytopenia, eczema, and recurrent infections (Wiskott-Aldrich syndrome) associated with milk antibodies, giant-cell pneumonia, and cytomegalic inclusion disease. Pediatrics 31:444–454
85. Orange JS, Stone KD, Turvey SE, Krzewski K (2004) The Wiskott-Aldrich syndrome. Cell Mol Life Sci 61(18):2361–2385
86. Ohya T, Yanagimachi M, Iwasawa K, Umetsu S, Sogo T, Inui A et al (2017) Childhood-onset inflammatory bowel diseases associated with mutation of Wiskott-Aldrich syndrome protein gene. World J Gastroenterol 23(48):8544–8552
87. Buchbinder D, Nugent DJ, Fillipovich AH (2014) Wiskott-Aldrich syndrome: diagnosis, current management, and emerging treatments. Appl Clin Genet 7:55–66
88. Sullivan KE, Mullen CA, Blaese RM, Winkelstein JA (1994) A multiinstitutional survey of the Wiskott-Aldrich syndrome. J Pediatr 125(6 Pt 1):876–885
89. McDonald-McGinn DM (2018) 22q11.2 deletion syndrome: a tiny piece leading to a big picture. Am J Med Genet A 176(10):2055–2057
90. Digilio MC, Giannotti A, Castro M, Colistro F, Ferretti F, Marino B et al (2003) Screening for celiac disease in patients with deletion 22q11.2 (DiGeorge/velo-cardio-facial syndrome). Am J Med Genet A 121A(3):286–288
91. Giardino G, Cirillo E, Maio F, Gallo V, Esposito T, Naddei R et al (2014) Gastrointestinal involvement in patients affected with 22q11.2 deletion syndrome. Scand J Gastroenterol 49(3):274–279
92. Markert ML, Sarzotti M, Ozaki DA, Sempowski GD, Rhein ME, Hale LP et al (2003) Thymus transplantation in complete DiGeorge syndrome: immunologic and safety evaluations in 12 patients. Blood 102(3):1121–1130
93. Digilio MC, Marino B, Bagolan P, Giannotti A, Dallapiccola B (1999) Microdeletion 22q11 and oesophageal atresia. J Med Genet 36(2):137–139
94. Kilic SS, Gurpinar A, Yakut T, Egeli U, Dogruyol H (2003) Esophageal atresia and tracheoesophageal fistula in a patient with Digeorge syndrome. J Pediatr Surg 38(8):E21–E23
95. Campbell IM, Sheppard SE, Crowley TB, McGinn DE, Bailey A, McGinn MJ et al (2018) What is new with 22q? An update from the 22q and You Center at the Children's Hospital of Philadelphia. Am J Med Genet A 176(10):2058–2069
96. Jackson O, Crowley TB, Sharkus R, Smith R, Jeong S, Solot C et al (2019) Palatal evaluation and treatment in 22q11.2 deletion syndrome. Am J Med Genet A 179(7):1184–1195
97. Humbert L, Cornu M, Proust-Lemoine E, Bayry J, Wemeau JL, Vantyghem MC et al (2018) Chronic mucocutaneous candidiasis in autoimmune polyendocrine syndrome type 1. Front Immunol 9:2570
98. D'Elios M, Baldari C, Annunziato F (2021) Cellular primary immunodeficiencies. Springer. https://doi.org/10.1007/978-3-030-70107-9

Index

A
ADAM17 deficiency, 111
Adenosine deaminase (ADA), 15
Antigen-presenting cells (APCs), 5
Artificial intelligence (AI), 49
Autoimmune enteropathy (AIE), 4, 6
Autoimmune polyendocrinopathy-candidiasis-ectodermal dystrophy (APECED) syndrome, 113

B
B-and T-cell receptors, 34, 35
Bayesian network (BN), 49
B-cell antigen-receptor (BCR), 11
B-cell epitope, 36, 37
B-cell receptors (BCRs), 35
Binary alignment map (BAM), 27
Biomarkers, 44

C
CBTOPE, 37
CD3 complex, 17
CD25 deficiency, 109
Chromatography, 41
Chronic granulomatous disease (CGD), 6, 7, 106, 107
Combined immunodeficiency (CID), 2
Common lymphoid progenitor (CLP), 11
CTLA4 insufficiency, 109

D
DiGeorge syndrome, 112, 113
DOCK8 Deficiency, 105
Dysregulation, 25

E
Electrospray ionization (ESI), 41
ElliPro, 37
Enzyme replacement therapy (ERT), 86
EPITOPIA, 37
Epstein-Barr virus, 104

G
Gene panel sequencing, 30
Gene regulation networks (GRNs), 40
Gene therapy, 44, 73, 84, 86
General data protection regulation (GDPR), 50
Genetic pleiotropism, 93, 94
Genome alignment, 27, 29
Graft-versus-host disease (GVHD), 70, 104
Gut-associated lymphoid tissue (GALT), 1, 3

H
Hematopoietic stem cells (HSCs), 74
Hematopoietic stem cells transplant (HSCT), 44, 67, 71, 84, 96
  complications, 73
  conditioning, 72
  donor type, 71
  gene therapy, 73, 74
  late effects, 73
HLA-Matching, 44, 45
Human Phenotype Ontology, 49
Hypomorphic mutations, 94

I
Immune dysregulation, 108
Inborn errors of immunity (IEI), 71, 93

M. M. D'Elios (ed.), *Severe Combined Immunodeficiency*, Rare Diseases of the Immune System, https://doi.org/10.1007/978-3-031-78864-2

Induced bronchus-associated lymphoid tissue (IBALT), 1
Inflammatory bowel disease (IBD), 2
Intravenous immune globulin (IVIG), 69
IPEX syndrome, 108, 109

J
JAK3 (Janus kinase 3) deficiency, 16, 81, 82

L
Late-onset combined immunodeficiency (LOCID), 91
LBtope, 36
Leukocyte adhesion deficiency type 1 (LAD-1), 108
LRBA deficiency, 110
Lymphocyte development, 11–13

M
Machine learning, 44
Major histocompatibility complex (MHC), 35
Mass spectrometry (MS), 41
Matched sibling donor (MSD), 85
Matched unrelated donor (MUD), 85
Metabolomics, 41
Metagenomics, 42
Motif matrices (MM), 35
Mucosa-associated lymphoid tissue (MALT), 1
Mucosal T cells, 3, 4
Multiple intestinal atresia (MIA), 2

N
Nasal-associated lymphoid tissue (NALT), 1
Natural killer (NK) cells, 11
Next-Generation Sequencing (NGS), 27
NFAT5 haploinsufficiency, 110

O
Omenn syndrome, 106

P
Patients with primary immunodeficiencies (PIDs), 113
Pneumocystis jirovecii pneumonia, 69, 80
Primary Immune Deficiency Treatment Consortium (PIDTC), 91, 92
Primary immunodeficiency (PID), 45
Protein druggability, 46
Proteomics, 41
Purine nucleoside phosphorylase (PNP), 83

Q
Quality control (QC), 40
Quantitative Affinity Matrices (QAMs), 35

R
Reactive oxygen species (ROS), 6
Reads alignment, 39
Recombination signal sequences (RSS), 16
Reticular dysgenesis (RD), 15, 83
RIPK1 deficiency, 110

S
Sanger sequencing, 26
Secretory immunoglobulin A (SIgA), 2
Severe combined immunodeficiency (SCID), 11, 12, 14, 67, 68, 70, 72, 73, 79, 91, 105
  diagnostic challenges, 95, 96
  genetic defects, 15–17
  lymphocyte development, 11–13
  mechanisms, 93, 94
  T lymphocytes, 11
  therapeutic approaches, 96
Single-cell isolation, 38
Single-cell RNA sequencing, 38
Structural bioinformatics, 34
Subcutaneous immune globulin (SCIG), 69
Support vector machines (SVM), 37
SVMtrip, 37

T
T cell receptor excision circle (TREC), 113
T-cell epitope prediction, 35
TGFB1 deficiency, 111
Thornton's method, 37

U
Uniform Manifold Approximation and Projection (UMAP), 40

V
Variants of uncertain significance (VUS), 95

W
Whole exome sequencing (WES), 32
Whole genome sequencing (WGS), 33
Wiskott-Aldrich syndrome (WAS), 112

X
XIAP deficiency, 111
X-linked severe combined immunodeficiency (X-SCID), 80

MIX
Papier aus verantwortungsvollen Quellen
Paper from responsible sources
FSC® C105338

If you have any concerns about our products,
you can contact us on
ProductSafety@springernature.com

In case Publisher is established outside the EU,
the EU authorized representative is:
Springer Nature Customer Service Center GmbH
Europaplatz 3, 69115 Heidelberg, Germany

Printed by Libri Plureos GmbH
in Hamburg, Germany